# HOSPITAL
# STAY
# HANDBOOK

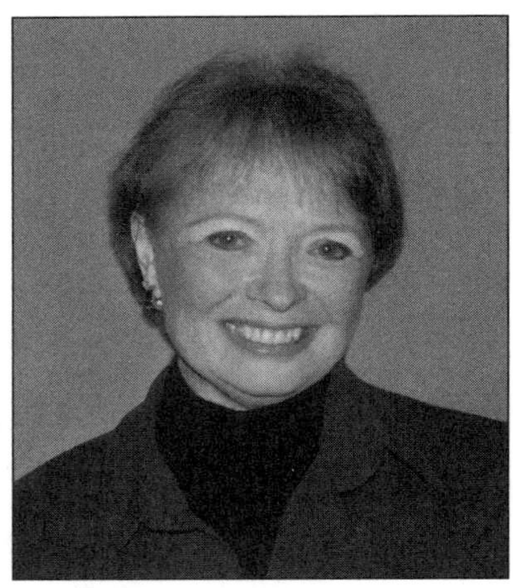

**About the Author**

Jari Holland Buck is a business consultant and trainer whose specialties include leadership and organizational development, transitions, and career enhancement. She founded her consulting group, now known as Majestic Wolf, in 1986. A medical layperson, Buck spent seven and a half months in four hospitals by the side of her critically ill husband. She dealt with hundreds of doctors and nurses and almost daily crises. This book represents the lessons she learned and used in partnership with the medical community to produce a miracle: her husband's survival.

# HOSPITAL STAY HANDBOOK

*A Guide to* **Becoming a Patient Advocate** *for Your* **Loved Ones**

**Jari Holland Buck**



Llewellyn Publications
Woodbury, Minnesota

First Edition
First Printing, 2007

Book design by Joanna Willis
Cover design by Ellen Dahl
Cover photograph © Ben Edwards / Corbis / PunchStock
Interior illustrations by Llewellyn art department

Reprint permissions appear on page 184.



**Library of Congress Cataloging-in-Publication Data**
Buck, Jari Holland.
[24/7 or Dead.]
Hospital stay handbook : a guide to becoming a patient advocate for your loved ones / Jari Holland Buck. — 1st ed.
p. cm.
"Previously published as *24/7 or Dead: A Handbook for Families with a Loved One in the Hospital* (AuthorHouse, Bloomington, Indiana) © 2005 by Jari Holland Buck."
Includes bibliographical references and index.
ISBN-13: 978-0-7387-1224-6
1. Patient advocacy—Handbooks, manuals, etc. 2. Hospital patients—Handbooks, manuals, etc. 3. Caregivers—Handbooks, manuals, etc. I. Title.
R727.45.B83 2007
610—dc22

2007030538



Llewellyn Publications
A Division of Llewellyn Worldwide, Ltd.
2143 Wooddale Drive, Dept. 978-0-7387-1224-6
Woodbury, MN 55125-2989, U.S.A.
www.llewellyn.com

Printed in the United States of America

## Important Note to the Reader

This book is dedicated to Bill Buck,
whose role in my life has completed the circle and brought me back to myself.

# CONTENTS

## FOR A DEEPER UNDERSTANDING

Foreword

# A DOCTOR'S PERSPECTIVE ON ADVOCACY: A VIEW FROM ABOVE THE BED

*Hospital Stay Handbook: A Guide to Becoming a Patient Advocate for Your Loved Ones* is written by a non-medical person—a regular American—who experienced firsthand the devastating events of her spouse's life-threatening illness. Jari Holland Buck knows upfront and personal the best and worst that can happen in a modern U.S. hospital today.

Her husband, Bill, was stricken suddenly with severe pancreatitis, which rapidly progressed to multiple organ failure, infection, seizures, and about every possible step toward death that any healthcare professional might imagine.

After more than seven months in the hospital—including six in ICUs on full life support—Bill is miraculously alive, walking, and recovering slowly from multiple long-term assaults on his system. That he is alive at all is a tribute to the wonders of modern medicine. But having been involved peripherally in Bill's hospital care and directly in Jari's journey with him, I can honestly say his survival is mostly due to Jari's committed presence. Her attention to detail, her willingness to question nurses, doctors, and therapists, and her insistence that they take her partnership seriously were key factors in his being alive today. She was tough. She asked hard questions. She insisted on being informed of all test results. I imagine she irritated some of the healthcare providers working so hard to keep Bill alive. But she was right to do so.

She was at Bill's side virtually every minute throughout all of his acute care, and it was good that she was. She picked up vital sign irregularities that could have led to death, despite continuous electronic monitoring. She collated information and asked probing questions. She sought the best care possible for Bill's complex and unique situation. When she did not get satisfactory answers, she insisted on more information, more explanation, and even a change of facilities and doctors. If she had not done these things, Bill surely would have died.

This book could only have been written by a family member determined to do the very best for a loved one. Healthcare professionals—unless they have been through such an intense and personal experience—cannot know in detail the emotional lives of those on the other side of the nurses' station.

As a doctor, I know I care about my patients and want to do my very best to help them. But there is no way I can ever be as diligent about every one of my patients as they themselves and their family will be. Thus, a partnership! If we doctors, nurses, therapists, and others in healthcare will take to heart Jari's and Bill's experiences and success, we can add an absolutely crucial dimension to our care of patients. We can never know everything, be aware of everything, or track every detail all of the time. We need help. Families and loved ones can truly help us in our journey to assist the lifesaving and healing processes to which we devote our lives. Let us invite them onto the healthcare team.

Jane Murray, MD
Sastun Center of Integrative Healthcare
Mission, Kansas
Former Director of the Division of Education
American Academy of Family Physicians
Past Chair of the Department of Family Medicine
University of Kansas Medical Center

# A PATIENT'S PERSPECTIVE ON ADVOCACY: A VIEW FROM THE BED

*Here is the test to find whether your mission on Earth is finished: if you're alive, it isn't.*
—Richard Bach, *Illusions*

My life changed forever the day my pancreas blew up. Although I am reasonably certain no doctor in the world would describe my disease in this fashion, that is how I think about it. I was an exercise fanatic and was convinced that if I worked out at least three times per week, I would be disease-proof. Obviously, that was a case of flawed thinking. Physically, I will never be whole again.

Before becoming disabled, I was rehabbing our home, building a scale railroad model, and filling the role of Chief Legal Counsel for an insurance company. My work frequently brought me in contact with doctors who, I believed, were entitled to obedience and respect on a nearly religious level. I now believe challenging a doctor could save your life. Mentally, I discovered the flaw in blind faith.

Prior to my illness, I did not understand how people could pray to a being I couldn't see, hear, touch, taste, or smell. I now recognize that prayer helped keep me alive. Spiritually, I can no longer dispute the power of joined hearts and minds in a quest for a miracle. I am one of those miracles!

I visited my surgeon last week for the first time in more than a year. I thanked him for saving my life. What was his response? "Your wife was the one who kept you alive." Once again my flawed thinking brought me up short. Emotionally, I live in debt and gratitude.



On every plane of my existence, my disease caused me to rethink suppositions and beliefs that I had carried with me throughout my life. The single most important shift I experienced happened when I observed and benefited from a form of fierce and protective energy wielded by my wife. Although it was sometimes embarrassing, sometimes amazing, sometimes humbling, I simply cannot deny the power of a dedicated, single-minded, caring advocate. I am fully convinced Jari is the reason I'm still here. Advocacy saved my life, and I would not have it any other way.

I am told Jari did a great deal of advocacy for me before I woke up, but I didn't see or hear her in action until the time I came to. My first conscious thought was, *Oh my God, I've been in a car wreck.* I panicked and got really scared. Following an explanation of my "dance with death," I began to watch the medical care providers, trying to determine whether I was being properly cared for.

What really got my attention was Jari. I noticed that doctors and other staff took Jari quite seriously, accepting her advice and even altering the course of care when she pointed out some aspects of my planned treatment that might have had a negative effect on me. She even got these busy professionals to pay attention to minor details such as my chapped lips and dry eyes.

My fondest memory of Jari's role and action was a phrase I overheard from just outside my room door: "If you think you've seen trouble before, you ain't seen nothin' yet!" Ordinarily, a family member would accept care plans and actions by medical staff without question or complaint. Jari did not respond that way ever, as far as I can tell. God bless her for that attitude.

There were very tough times when Jari needed to be the cool head in the group. On one occasion during a holiday, I needed an immediate consultation but a staff person refused to call an MD at his home "because he was entitled to time with his family, too." Jari kicked some serious butt that day, and I got what

I needed. Perhaps I even got to stay alive because she had the guts to call protocol into question. Nice talk and good manners don't save lives. As an attorney, I am professionally trained to speak up on behalf of another, but I learned some lessons from Jari.

Know what ails your loved one. Use the Internet to find the information that is there for the taking. You can even begin to talk like a "real doctor" and be compellingly persuasive in the process. My wife got the equivalent of a PhD in medicine through her extensive study of all my conditions. And if there is a way to feel in touch and in balance while a loved one is battling for life, it is through such self-initiated study and challenge to the status quo. I believe this is the one time in your life to make sure you are heard, even though the listener may not want to hear what you have to say. Kick butt and don't try to make friends. You and your loved one are in a pitched battle to make sure that life and health prevail.

William C. Buck, JD

# AN ADVOCATE'S PERSPECTIVE ON ADVOCACY: A VIEW FROM THE BEDSIDE

*Only a person who risks is free.*
*The pessimist complains about the wind;*
*The optimist expects it to change;*
*And the realist adjusts the sails.*
—William Arthur Ward, *To Risk*

The very best place for a critically ill patient is in the hospital. The very worst place for a critically ill patient is in the hospital.

It is a double bind of the worst kind, especially for family members of that critically ill patient. Hospitals have become such frightening places for a variety of reasons. Let's begin by looking at the economic factors that affect the cost and quality of care.

Over the next twenty years, those of us who are baby boomers will strain an already ailing system as we enter our senior years and require additional care, adding 76 to 78 million potential patients in that time frame.[1]

1 William D. Novelli, "Beyond Fifty: America's Future," speech given at the City Club of Cleveland, July 20, 2001, http://www.aarp.org/about_aarp/aarp_leadership/on_issues/aging_issues/a2002-12-31-novellicleveland.html.

Out-of-pocket healthcare costs are skyrocketing for all Americans, especially those with low incomes and fixed-income retirees. These people cannot earn more to offset the accelerating costs, and as a result they forego medicines and treatment, compromising their health. Today, out-of-pocket healthcare costs average 19 percent of income for people 65 and over and almost 50 percent for those on Medicare.[2]

Health insurance premiums paid by working employees have increased 73 percent since 2000, at a rate five times faster than workers' earnings have risen. For the typical Fortune 500 company, the expense of employee health insurance will zero out profits soon if nothing changes.[3] Employees and employers face tough decisions inside a healthcare system that is primarily employment-based. The eighteen-month cap on COBRA benefits offered to departing employees only compounds the problem. More and more workers are either losing coverage, opting for catastrophic coverage only, or dropping healthcare insurance altogether as a way of managing costs. The number of uninsured has grown by more than one million people per year for the last five years.[4] This trend leads to later treatment of sicker people at higher, nonreimbursed costs.

Among industrialized nations, the United States spends more than twice the average per-capita amount on healthcare. But the quality of that care does not parallel the extra spending. These facts were noted in a Commonwealth Fund report published online in September 2006:

- As a whole, the United States healthcare system falls short of the benchmarks set by other industrialized nations, scoring just 66 points out of 100. As a result, 150,000 lives are lost and $50 billion to $100 billion are needlessly spent each year.
- Preventive care, too, is underperforming, with only about half of U.S. residents receiving the recommended care. This lack results in the onset of dis-

2 Ibid.

3 National Coalition on Health Care, "Health Insurance Cost," National Coalition on Health Care, http://www.nchc.org/facts/cost.shtml.

4 Steven Reinberg, "U.S. Health-Care System Scores a D for Quality," *HealthDay News*, Sept. 20, 2006, http://www.medicinenet.com/script/main/art.asp?articlekey=64267.

eases and conditions that could have been avoided or at least delayed. Type 2 diabetes is just one example.

- The United States ranks near the bottom on life expectancy and last on infant mortality. Access to healthcare is unequal, often varying with factors such as income and racial or ethnic group.
- U.S. healthcare costs are higher per capita than in nations such as Canada that have universal coverage, ensuring coverage for all. Inefficiencies and duplication of services are part of the problem, as illustrated by the slow adoption of electronic medical record systems in the United States.[5]



What does all this add up to for us as healthcare consumers? Care that is not optimal when measured against international standards, provided unequally at ever-increasing cost, and aimed at treatment rather than prevention!

Economics aside, the more distressing reason for poor healthcare is the loss of the concept of care. The *American Heritage Dictionary* defines care as "attentive assistance or treatment to those in need."[6] Today, providing medical services to consumers is a business—a business that, to the uneducated and the educated alike, seems not to care at all about the human factors involved in the treatment of the body and the spirit.

My husband was hospitalized for seven and a half months, six of which were in intensive care and on life support. My motivation in sharing our experience is not driven by a desire to lambaste managed care providers or to indict medical insurance companies. Anyone who remembers how medical treatment was provided just ten or twenty years ago can only be disappointed with the services provided today. The healthcare system in the United States today is badly broken and I, as a consumer, do not know how to fix it.

Given this healthcare environment, every patient runs extreme risks—in part due to the low level of the type of care that has been historically provided by nurses. In the spirit of cost containment, hospitals are notoriously understaffed.

---

5 Ibid.

6 *The American Heritage Dictionary of the English Language*, 4th ed., s.v. "care."

I have personally witnessed a 1:16 nurse-to-patient ratio. How can any human being, even with the best intentions, provide anything beyond the most basic physical care to sixteen patients? For care partners (formerly known as nurses' aides), the ratio can be even more lopsided.

A University of Pennsylvania study of 232,000 surgical patients at 168 hospitals concluded that a patient's overall risk of death rose roughly 7 percent with each additional patient (above four) assigned to the same nurse's care.[7] So, for example, on the day my husband experienced a 1:16 nurse-to-patient ratio, he was 84 percent more likely to die.



The same study identified such ratios as a cause of job burnout and dissatisfaction among nurses. And the consequences add up to a critical nursing shortage, a problem that is only growing. The Health Resources and Services Administration (HRSA) projects a shortage of one million nurses by 2020.[8] The U.S. Bureau of Labor Statistics projects the same shortage by 2012.[9] Either way, U.S. hospitals are in trouble. What is behind this nursing shortage? The factors include:

- Short staffing and work environment. Between 1980 and 2000, nursing ranks shrank by 20 percent because of mandatory overtime, overwork due to staffing shortages and rising patient counts, increased stress, lack of support from hospital management, and other factors affecting the quality of work life.[10]

---

7 Linda H. Aiken et al., "Hospital Nurse Staffing and Patient Mortality, Nurse Burnout, and Job Dissatisfaction," *Journal of the American Medical Association* 288, no. 16 (Oct. 23, 2002), http://jama.ama-assn.org/cgi/content/full/288/16/1987.

8 U.S. Department of Health and Human Services, Health Resources and Services Administration (HRSA), "What Is Behind HRSA's Projected Supply, Demand, and Shortage of Registered Nurses?", HRSA Bureau of Health Professions, http://bhpr.hrsa.gov/healthworkforce/reports/behindrnprojections/index.htm.

9 American Association of Colleges of Nursing, "With Enrollments Rising for the 5th Consecutive Year, U.S. Nursing Schools Turn Away More Than 30,000 Qualified Applications in 2005," http://www.aacn.nche.edu/Media/NewsReleases/2005/enrl05.htm.

10 Susan Jacoby, "The Nursing Squeeze," *AARP Bulletin*, May 2003.

- Job dissatisfaction, even among young nurses. Overall, more than 40 percent of hospital nurses reported dissatisfaction with their jobs. Among those under 30, one out of three was planning a job change in the next year, according to a study released in the *Journal of the American Medical Association*.[11]

- Low pay. Pay is directly tied to the number of nurses found in hospital settings. As pay stays flat, more nurses choose less stressful environments such as doctors' offices.[12]

- An aging and retiring workforce. Nurses are baby boomers, too, and one survey reported that 55 percent of nurses plan to retire between 2011 and 2020.[13] Their average age is rising, too: it was 46.8 in March 2004.[14]

- Fewer nurses entering the profession. Nursing schools turned away 32,617 qualified applicants in 2005.[15]



So what does this mean for us? Lower quality of care, longer emergency room wait times, cancelled elective surgeries due to short staffing, greater likelihood of mistakes, older nurses with heavier patient loads. Clearly, things are not getting better. In fact, understaffing is already affecting patient outcomes. Since 1996, 24 percent of hospitals' reports of patient deaths and injuries were affected by

---

11 U.S. Department of Health and Human Services, Health Resources and Services Administration (HRSA), "HRSA Responds to the Nursing Shortage: Results from the 2003 Nursing Scholarship Program and the Nursing Education Loan Repayment Program, 2002–2003," HRSA Bureau of Health Professions, http://bhpr.hrsa.gov/nursing/2003NELRPNSPRTC/Chapter2.htm.

12 American Federation of State, County and Municipal Employees, "Low Nurse Wages and Nurse Shortages: Cause and Effect," http://www.afscme.org/publications/10951.cfm.

13 American Association of Colleges of Nursing (AACN), "Fact Sheet: Nursing Shortage," March 2007, http://www.aacn.nche.edu/Media/FactSheets/NursingShortage.htm.

14 U.S. Department of Health and Human Services, Health Resources and Services Administration (HRSA), "Preliminary Findings: 2004 National Sample Survey of Registered Nurses," HRSA Bureau of Health Professions, http://bhpr.hrsa.gov/healthworkforce/reports/rnpopulation/preliminaryfindings.htm.

15 The American Association of Colleges of Nursing, "With Enrollments Rising for the 5th Consecutive Year, U.S. Nursing Schools Turn Away More Than 30,000 Qualified Applications in 2005," http://www.aacn.nche.edu/Media/NewsReleases/2005/enrl05.htm.

low nursing staff levels, according to a report from the Joint Commission (formerly known as JCAHO, the Joint Commission on Accreditation of Healthcare Organizations).[16]

What about doctors? Today, many doctors are severely overworked because the only way they can cover their expenses is to take on additional patients. Why? Because insurance carriers have created the concept of preferred providers, thereby enabling them to heavily discount doctors' fees (up to 50 percent). The result is that doctors need to treat up to twice the number of patients they previously treated to achieve the same financial return. Additionally, Medicare is not keeping up with the rising cost of healthcare, leading many doctors to refuse to treat Medicare patients.

And then there are the hospital administrators, who are driven by the numbers as surely as any CEO in the private sector.

Those who work in the U.S. healthcare system see these problems every day, of course. But people within a system, even when they hate the system, are often reluctant to change it—a human fact I have seen countless times in my work as an organizational consultant. With the status quo, at least people know how to operate and respond. Anything new requires a new behavior. And that takes extra effort, something most healthcare providers find almost impossible, given the stress of their daily workloads. Although most of them might agree in principle that the system needs changing, that new behaviors are needed, they may naturally resist change. But as healthcare consumers and patient advocates, we can push for change, push for that extra effort, and get better care—even in the current healthcare setting.

That is the subject of this book. Through my own story as a patient advocate—often painful but always educational—this book illustrates many of the flaws and dangers of our healthcare system and shows how to navigate it as safely as possible. Changing the system feels overwhelming and impossible. So let's assume the status quo and focus on protecting our loved ones and ourselves. We can do this by taking personal responsibility for minimizing the risks

16 U.S. Department of Health and Human Services, Health Resources and Services Administration (HRSA), "HRSA Responds to the Nursing Shortage."

to the patient due to inadequate care. How do we do this? By adding another layer of care: by coordinating and/or providing bedside advocacy twenty-four hours a day, seven days a week. Of course, advocates needn't exhaust themselves into burnout, ignoring their own needs. Share the responsibility among several people, as many as necessary for the sake of everyone's health. But I do strongly recommend the full-time presence of a family member or friend for every patient in a hospital. I had no previous experience doing this. But as I plunged ahead, I learned some very important lessons about what it took to keep my husband alive.

What does advocacy look like? Many advocates have gone before us, and we can learn from them. Patient advocacy is supported by AARP (formerly known as the American Association of Retired Persons) and the National Patient Safety Foundation (NPSF). The first part of this book is tactical, outlining fourteen key recommendations for patients and their advocates. In many cases these are lessons I learned the hard way. The second part of this book discusses advocacy and caregiving from a philosophical perspective; it also offers guidance on handling the financial matters that often accompany medical care. In the "Lessons in Advocacy" section you will find the NPSF's "Consumer Fact Sheet: The Role of the Patient Advocate," reprinted with permission. The NPSF website, and the others recommended in this book's "Resources" section, will provide you with more tools and knowledge to help you step into this new role.

A good first step into advocacy is to set your intention. In my own spiritual practice, how I do what I do is not nearly as important as setting my intention clearly and simply. Intention then drives every subsequent step I take on behalf of my patient. When healthcare workers are faced with a committed person's intention, they understand. They may not like it, but they understand. Their response may be very different when faced with a challenge that is not grounded in intention: in my case, the best interests of the patient. After all, how can healthcare workers object to what is in the patient's best interest? That is their job. When in doubt about what to do, lead with your intention.

Follow your intention by educating yourself, acting with courage, taking risks, and collaborating with family, friends, and healthcare providers—all in service of full-time advocacy. Without the full-time presence of an advocate for every patient in a hospital, I believe there is a very good chance mistakes will be made. Some of these mistakes could cost your loved one his or her life or health. Remember what the statistics showed us: U.S. healthcare is not optimal, it is provided unequally at ever-increasing costs, and it is aimed at treatment rather than prevention. Its systemic problems result in a greater likelihood of mistakes, poor staff-to-patient ratios, longer emergency room wait times, cancelled elective surgeries due to short staffing, and so on. These are the very issues we must prepare to address and prevent on behalf of our patient.

Please join me as an advocate at the bedside. Let your heart and mind be filled with this simple intention: "everything in the best interest of my patient." Remember, we do this for love.

Jari Holland Buck

# READ ME FIRST, READ ME OFTEN: HOW TO USE THIS BOOK

*I will hold open a space for you in the world and allow your right to fill it with authentic vocation and purpose. For as long as your search takes, you have my loyalty.*
—Theodore Roszak

If you have found your way to this book, it is likely that you or a loved one is either in the hospital or facing hospitalization in the near future.

When we are ill, we are probably not at our best. When a loved one is ill, we are probably not at our best at first, either. When I became a patient advocate for my husband Bill—not a role I had planned for—I found myself highly distractible and nervous at first, with a very short attention span. There was so much to learn, so quickly, and stakes were so high.

This book will help ground you. It will give you the practical tools to truly do your best as an advocate, ensuring your loved one gets the care that is needed and deserved. It also offers some spiritual tools and approaches. The first part of this book provides fourteen recommendations. You will learn what problems to anticipate and how to help prevent them, to weave the practical and the spiritual, success and failure, life and death, joy and sadness. All of these concepts live on a continuum, as does the care your patient receives. Since the practical is what drives most of us to seek this information, I begin there. However, as fear and anxiety take their toll, the spiritual begins to take on a much larger role. Once you have the basics in place, seek support more broadly: see this book's Resources section for helpful organizations, publications, and other tools.

Here's how to use the information in this book:

- Read each recommendation.
- Decide which recommendations are most relevant to your situation. For example, Recommendation 2, "Choose Your Hospital with Awareness" may be less relevant if your loved one is already hospitalized, or if your options are very limited. Still, it is worth your time to read: you will learn what qualities to look for in your current hospital, what problems you might anticipate, and how to help minimize them.
- Pick one recommendation and try it. Avoid trying to do them all at once. You might overwhelm yourself, lose confidence, and possibly compromise your working relationships with professional care providers. Absorb one recommendation fully, and take your time.
- Have confidence and take the time to learn. You can do this! Anything you can face, you can handle. Remember, you are learning a brand-new language and brand-new skills. Ask questions over and over until you understand. Take notes. Be gentle with yourself.
- Now add another recommendation. You may find that the order here makes sense, but if you want to tackle them in a different order, do it. The issue is not the order, but your choice of the recommendations that are most helpful and relevant to your situation.
- Use the checklists that appear in several of the recommendations. They will help you keep a clear head. Feel free to adapt them as needed.
- Expand your sphere of influence courageously. Listen to yourself, and risk taking action when control isn't possible. You cannot plan and control everything. You cannot always expect clear goals and measurable progress. But

you can maintain clear values. Whatever has already occurred, it is behind you and cannot be changed. Focus on what can be and must be.

- Keep your eyes and heart open. In the midst of it all, there will be moments of exquisite joy.

"Only the truth that is genuinely experienced on all levels of being . . . has the power to change a human being," said Rollo May.[1] Be prepared to be personally changed by what you are about to read and experience. The world of healthcare has changed and is still changing. We must adapt to that reality. Even with the best intentions, in the current system, healthcare providers have feet of clay. We may be medical laypeople, but we must use our newfound knowledge and our personal power, fearlessly standing up for our patient's best interests.



In the words of Rich Work:

If I can keep you in these Laws,
If I can keep you in these Fears,
If I can keep you in this Power,
If I can keep you from Loving yourself—
Just one of these—I can control you.
All of them—I can own you.[2]

We cannot allow someone else to make our healthcare decisions; we must act as partners. To do that, join me in learning the laws, working through the fears, recognizing the power of partnership, loving yourself and your family, maximizing your influence in important decisions, and owning your desire for health, happiness, and life itself.

At times during Bill's hospitalization, I was afraid to speak up. Sometimes I allowed busy care providers to make me feel like a bother, or "less than worthy" to ask questions. But I was emboldened by these words of Eleanor Roosevelt: "There is no more liberating, no more exhilarating experience than to determine

1 Rollo May, *Existential Psychology* (New York: Random House, 1988), 13–14.

2 Rich Work with Ann Marie Goth, *Awaken to the Healer Within* (Mosinee, WI: Asini Publishing, 1995), 153.

one's position, state it bravely, and then act boldly. Action creates its own courage; and courage is as contagious as fear."[3] And God knows, there was plenty of fear. I needed another compelling emotion to salve my heart.

We don't take this medical journey by choice. But it might change us; it might teach us about ourselves. Before my husband, Bill, got pancreatitis, he described himself as bulletproof. He worked out three times a week. Death was not on his agenda, not ever. He couldn't stand the smell of lilies because it reminded him of funerals. An attorney, he refused to execute a will or any healthcare directives: he didn't want to think about the possibility of death. I, on the other hand, was overacquainted with death. During my childhood I buried seven family members and friends in five years.



I laugh in retrospect when I think of this match made out of "death aversion." By running away from it, we became a powerful magnet for death. Bill is still alive. But death did find us, hiding in the darkness of my memories and his denial. We did experience death, as nothing will ever be the same again.

Your journey will be different from ours. But the fourteen recommendations in this book should serve you well. How do I know? They are my own hardwon lessons, learned through experience. Before turning to those recommendations, I invite you to hear, in brief, the story that "credentialed" me as a patient advocate. If you have time, retrace with me the journey my husband, the patient, and I, the advocate, traveled from catastrophic illness to recovery.

If you do not have time, or if the illness or injury at hand requires immediate action, your next step is to read the recommendations, select one, and begin. Godspeed in your endeavor.

3 Eleanor Roosevelt, *Tomorrow Is Now* (New York: Harper, 1963).

### Our Story

# ONE DAY, AFTER LUNCH

*God does not send us despair in order to kill us;*
*He sends it in order to awaken us to new life.*
—Hermann Hesse, *Reflections*

I have found that stories, especially real-life stories, have power. The cross-cultural anthropologist Angeles Arrien calls storytelling one of the "healing salves . . . It has long been recognized that . . . [stories] return to us the qualities of wonder, hope and awe."[1] Bill and I have a story, and here it is. Believe me when I say we have been there.

One day, after a vigorous noon-hour workout at the local health club, my husband, Bill, returned to his office, munching on a tuna-salad sandwich. About thirty minutes later, he walked into his friend Skip's office and asked for a Rolaid, complaining of a stomachache. Thirty minutes after that, he collapsed on the floor in excruciating pain; paramedics were summoned. I am told the pain of acute pancreatitis is comparable to childbirth, but I get ahead of myself . . .

After the 911 call, Skip called me. I am a consultant and work from home. On that particular day I was at my computer, working intently on an analysis of

1 Angeles Arrien, *The Four-Fold Way: Walking the Paths of the Warrior, Teacher, Healer and Visionary* (San Francisco: HarperSanFrancisco, 1993).

employee interview data and, frankly, had not even showered or dressed. I was still in my pajamas from the previous night. The date was October 23, 2000, a day I will never forget, as it marked the commencement of a trip into hell that I feared we would never survive.



It was about 2:10 when I got Skip's call. He told me not to panic, but wanted me to know the paramedics were transporting Bill to the hospital. Because this was an emergency situation, he was taken to the hospital closest to his workplace.

Bill had five of the signs of a medical emergency as defined by the American College of Emergency Physicians: (1) difficulty in breathing or shortness of breath, (2) chest or abdominal pain or pressure, (3) fainting, (4) sudden dizziness, and (5) sudden, severe pain.[2]

Although Bill was in severe pain, he was conscious and talking while being loaded into the ambulance. Skip told me Bill had asked him not to call me: he didn't want to worry me. Bill knew, of course, about the many family member deaths during my younger years, and my terror of a repeat episode. Skip obviously ignored this request and called me anyway.

I thought it couldn't be that serious if Bill was still conscious, so I took the time to finish my interrupted thought about the employee data before I saved the file. Boy, was that a mistaken assumption.

At 2:18 I showered, threw on some clothes and drove quickly to meet Skip and another of Bill's colleagues in front of his office. Since I did not know where Bill had been taken, I followed them in my car to the nearest hospital. As I came to expect, the hospital required me to provide insurance information before I was allowed access to my husband.

Bill was sitting on an emergency room bed, doubled over in terrible pain. The staff X-rayed his abdomen, drew blood, and did a CT scan. Then they placed a tube down his throat to drain and remove the contents of his stomach. His pain would be eased when that was done, they promised, but relief was not forthcoming.

2 American College of Emergency Physicians, "When Should I Go to the Emergency Department?", http://www.acep.org/webportal/PatientsConsumers/HealthSubjectsByTopic/emcare/whentogotoed.htm.

The emergency room (ER) doctor frequently stopped by to speak with us, and told me he had asked for a consultation with a specialist. When the specialist arrived, he asked me—and Bill, who could not speak through the pain—how much alcohol Bill typically consumed. I replied he was not a drinker. The doctor repeated the question, apparently not believing me. I replied, "About six beers in a banner year." He then asked me if I knew for certain, adding that many drunks are good at hiding their drinking.

Having earlier experienced alcoholism and recovery in my own family, I was aware of this. As a result, Bill and I had discussed alcohol use before venturing into our relationship some fourteen years earlier. So when the doctor asked again about Bill's alcohol use, my patience ran out for the first of several hundred times to come. I stepped in close and told the doctor forcefully that I knew for a fact Bill was not a closet drinker. I had now answered his question for the third and last time and we were *not* going to discuss it again! Little did I know that I would be asked this question thirty more times over the course of Bill's illness: alcoholism is the number one cause of his disease.

The doctor finally apologized, explaining that Bill had acute pancreatitis and would be hospitalized for several days. No food or water by mouth would be allowed until his pancreas calmed down. I later learned that all the medical community knows to do for pancreatitis is to maintain the patient while the disease runs its course.

Let's call this facility "Hospital A" to distinguish it from the three others to come. Hospital A admitted Bill to its intensive care unit (ICU), hooked him up to several monitors, and provided a morphine pump to self-administer pain medication.

One of the monitors to which Bill was connected measured how much oxygen was getting to his body. When the oxygen level was too low, an alarm would sound. I stayed in Bill's hospital room that night and the alarm went off some forty times. In spite of my coaching him to breathe deeply, he was clearly not getting enough oxygen. The next morning, about fifteen hours after admission, the same specialist told me that to ensure Bill got enough air, we needed to temporarily place him on a ventilator, a machine that forcibly delivers humidified air under pressure to a patient's lungs. This temporary solution lasted six months.

Bill and I both said, "I love you," and a nurse asked me to leave the room as the process could be "upsetting" for family members to watch. Bill was anesthetized into unconsciousness to ease the placement of the tube down his throat, which connected him with the ventilator. The doctors were still advising me a five- to seven-day stay was probable.

Over the course of the next week, Bill's condition continued to deteriorate. His breathing, even on the ventilator, grew so bad that when the staff had to transport him down one floor for tests, he desaturated: his oxygen consumption fell far below acceptable levels.

Nurses drew blood at least daily to determine what was going on metabolically. More and more tubes were placed into my unconscious husband: intravenous ones ("IV lines") to deliver medicines—drugs I did not yet understand—and other lines to hydrate and nourish his body.

In those early days, my focus was on what had caused this to happen to a perfectly healthy human being. My brother-in-law researched acute pancreatitis on the Internet, and my sister delivered the printed results daily when she visited. During his seven months of hospitalization, we explored and discounted every causal agent of his disease. To this day, Bill is one of the 15 percent of documented pancreatitis patients whose illness was idiopathic: cause unknown.

Skip and Bill's boss came to Hospital A daily and sat with me for hours. Bill's employer dispatched the company jet to Florida to fly Bill's mother to the airport closest to the hospital; his children's air travel was also covered. The company even covered all of their hotel expenses. I came to understand that those emloyed by his organization—among many others—did not expect him to survive.

Bill's prognosis worsened. During the second week, for the first of four times, Bill "coded": short for code blue, the hospital special-response code for a heart or breathing stoppage. His ventilator tube got plugged with mucus and he stopped breathing. Thanks to his nurse's rapid response and the coordinated efforts of his respiratory therapist, he survived.

Now the doctors were saying Bill might have ARDS—adult respiratory distress syndrome—and one speculated that he might also have congestive heart failure. So I researched both of those conditions.

During the third week, Bill had his first of thirteen episodes of sepsis: a blood infection that in his case was usually caused by an infection in an IV line. Over the course of four hours, his blood pressure dropped repeatedly to 60/30. We could raise it to 80/40 only for very short periods of time. The nursing staff administered a series of drugs called pressors, designed to elevate blood pressure, yet his pressure still hovered at a deathlike level.

When they started the third pressor, called Levophed (Levo for short), the nurses were considerate enough to withhold the informal remarks that typically accompany Levo—"leave 'em dead with Levophed" and "dread phed." Nurses and doctors have enough experience with this drug to know that most patients who receive it do not survive. I was informed that Levo virtually clamps off the blood supply to the patient's hands and feet. A potential result might be the amputation of Bill's fingers or toes—if he survived. And that was a big if, I later learned. My response was, "What choice do I have? Go ahead."

That evening, one of the nurses took my head in her hands and told me, "Bill may go to God tonight." My sister Sue and Skip stayed with me all night, alternately holding my hand and Bill's. I whispered in his ear that if he needed to leave, I would try to understand, but I really wanted him to stay.

We went through twenty-four vials of a pressure-enhancing medication, at one point having it delivered by emergency courier from a nearby hospital. Sometime after midnight, Bill stabilized. When a suspicious-looking ART (arterial) line was removed the following morning, it turned out to be infected.

Within twenty-four hours of this first sepsis, his kidneys failed (acute kidney failure), his liver failed (shock liver), and his blood stopped clotting (disseminated intravascular coagulation, or DIC). The doctors also suspected Bill had suffered a heart attack during sepsis: his body showed evidence of an elevated heart enzyme level that typically follows myocardial episodes. Subsequently, I discovered he had suffered a stroke during this episode as well!

My research was producing statistics showing probable recovery for each of his organ failures and things had statistically moved well into the "probably will not survive this" realm. We were now in multi-organ failure syndrome—a very bad thing.

By this time, Bill was on a rotating bed: a bed whose position can be shifted to reduce the chance of bedsores, and it can also improve breathing. Bill's color was that of the maroon fabric covering the bed. A dermatologist examined him to determine if the skin color was a result of sepsis or a drug reaction. Although there was no drug reaction, from that point on, Bill wore a wristband warning of a possible allergy to a very powerful antibiotic.

The doctors soon started him on kidney dialysis, which frequently dropped his blood pressure to a terrifyingly low level. They transfused him during dialysis to help his clotting factors, and we waited with crossed fingers to see if his liver function would return.

The following week brought his second sepsis episode, every bit as critical as the first. But this time, we did not have to turn to the drug of last resort, Levophed. I found small comfort in that fact when I learned that he again had an infected ART line and, in all probability, had suffered another stroke. At that time, I thought it was the first stroke. Moreover, within twenty-four hours of this sepsis, Bill had two seizures while receiving dialysis. These seizures occurred when I was away from Hospital A for the first time since his illness began. I'm surprised I wasn't killed in an automobile accident as I raced back to the hospital after receiving word of his condition.

I was terrified during the neurological consult after the seizures, as the specialist explained all the possible causes and effects. Stroke damage, dead brain tissue, and brain damage were in play for several days while we awaited test results. We never did learn specifically what caused his seizures. In my research I discovered that they could have been caused by any one of the ten or so conditions from which Bill was suffering. He was placed on anti-seizure medication for about a month, after which it was discontinued ("d/c'd" in medical lingo) with no consequences.

Meanwhile, I had essentially moved into Bill's area of Hospital A. Two sleeping rooms with an adjoining bathroom were available to family members. I had occupied one of them since his third day there. I also shut down my consulting practice so I could be at the hospital full time.

During the rare bedside moments that were uneventful, I read about each catastrophe from material off the Internet. I also began asking questions of and noting answers from the doctors, identifying my source of information as online articles and texts. I requested explanations about everything—how to read the monitors, what they measured, how to read his lab results, what they meant, how equipment in his room worked, what each line and drug was for, what each procedure was designed to test or accomplish, and on and on and on. I decided I wanted to know and understand as much as I could, since praying and hand-holding seemed to be all I could otherwise do.



Bill had tons of visitors, a practice I soon had to stop. Bill was unconscious, and we were both well beyond the point where visitors could comfort us. I always found myself recounting the most recent crises to these well-meaning people, resulting in more stress and anguish to me. Our primary care doctor had begun visiting us at the hospital, and I asked her for antidepressant and anti-anxiety drugs. Frankly, at times my anti-anxiety medication was the only thing that kept me in my body.

The next weeks passed in a blur of tests, continuing sepsis, raging infections, fevers up to 105°, anemia, pneumonia, and ileus (he stopped having bowel movements). The hospital also had an apparent power outage that was heart-stopping (to me, the respiratory therapist, and Bill's nurse). During a circuit change, the maintenance crew had forgotten to inform the ICU staff to stand by while their equipment switched over to emergency backup power. Fortunately, Bill's care providers were on the ball and came at a run, ready to manually bag him—push air into his lungs with a specially designed breathing bag—should the emergency power fail to kick on, thereby putting the ventilator out of commission. This experience taught me at a gut level the value of the electrical outlets with red-colored plates. These plates indicate electrical circuits linked to emergency backup power. Obviously, critical equipment such as ventilators are plugged into red-plated outlets.

Bill's breathing difficulties continued, closely watched by his pulmonologist—a doctor who specializes in the lungs. The pulmonologist advised a tracheotomy was necessary: a surgical incision in the neck that gives direct access to the airway. In this case, it would prevent damage to his voice box that could result from the lengthy presence of a breathing tube down his throat. When the doctors prepared Bill for the trach, they discovered he was "one in a million"—a vein ran right across the proposed trach site. This discovery delayed the trach procedure and terrified me because, should the specialist performing the trach hit the vein, Bill might bleed to death. The team consulted a thoracic surgeon: a specialist who conducts surgery on the chest. That surgeon ultimately oversaw the procedure, which was finally performed without a hitch.

This was the first of many times I was told, "Your husband's condition is one in a million." I came to associate those words with only the smallest chance for survival.

In extreme acute pancreatitis cases—of which Bill's was one—pancreatic pseudocysts often develop in the abdomen. Pseudocysts contain free-floating pieces of dead pancreatic tissue surrounded by liquid, blood, and potentially, pus. The doctors suspected that during his seven weeks at Hospital A, Bill had developed one of these and that it had burst, causing another septic episode.

He ultimately developed four pseudocysts. Since the staff at Hospital A were uncertain about the next course of treatment, they suggested that when—if—Bill's condition improved, I could move him to one of two hospitals with more experience treating his problem. One of these—Hospital B—was out of state; the other was local.

Hospital B was well known for treating only the most critically ill, and Bill certainly qualified. On December 12, Bill was airlifted there by a LifeFlight helicopter. I will never forget seeing him strapped to a stretcher on the tarmac, attached to a ventilator, pale as death, but with eyes wide open in anticipation of flying. Bill loves to fly, and even sick and drugged, he had some awareness of his surroundings. As we lifted off, I prayed I would bring Bill back from this consult alive, but I feared he would return in a body bag.

Upon arrival at the new facility, Bill promptly went septic again. However, unlike the previous one, Hospital B initially barred me from his ICU room (a practice that was eventually changed). Over the next ten ugly days, his earlier diagnosis was totally rejected until the specialists at this facility could confirm it for themselves. In the meantime, Bill was poked, prodded, X-rayed, CT scanned, bled, and needle-aspirated: a doctor withdrew liquid from his abdomen through a long needle to determine the contents of the pseudocyst. The doctors' diagnosis was essentially this: "There is nothing we can do for your husband. If we cut him open, he will die. Take him home and let him die peacefully."

During Bill's stay at Hospital B, he was denied critical treatment (dialysis), which necessitated a cardioversion (electric clappers attached to the chest) when his heart rate exceeded 160 beats a minute for about an hour's time. He was also denied medically necessary equipment (a rotating bed) and soon developed first-stage pressure wounds (bedsores, stage 1 of 3). Meanwhile, I struggled to gain access to his room, his records, and his lab and test results, all of which I needed in order to be an informed healthcare partner.



After ten days Bill was airlifted out of there, and I heaved an immense sigh of relief. This time he was admitted to Hospital C. It was in the same city as Hospital A, so Bill picked up the same three primary physicians who had previously worked with him. Now he was more likely to have round-the-clock doctor availability. For the next ten days, however, Bill's condition continued to deteriorate. (I always wondered if that was possible, given all he had already experienced.) On January 12, I was informed his pseudocysts were no longer sterile but had become infected. Surgery was now a necessity, not an option. This time I was told, "If we do *not* cut him open, he will die." Reflecting on the diagnosis of the world-class experts at the previous hospital—"If we cut him open, he will die"—this sounded like a certain-to-die situation. The surgery could not be done at Hospital C, however. Recognizing I would probably be moving him to his last living space, I had to choose between two locations for surgery: Hospital B, from which we had recently returned, and Hospital D, a local teaching hospital.

I had been wondering whether I had made a mistake transporting Bill to Hospital B in the first place—until I was faced with this choice. Had I chosen Hospital B for the surgery, I now believed it would have killed him: we were lucky that we had learned not to trust that facility. So the only choice was Hospital D, our local option.

Ambulance service was arranged, and once again I moved Bill. Bill was now sixty pounds lighter than on the day he was first admitted to the hospital. As a result of a condition called ascites, his waistline was so enlarged that he looked like he was fifteen months pregnant with triplets. He was still unconscious, still on full life support, still on daily kidney dialysis, and still receiving massive blood transfusions. He was also being nourished with a feeding tube inserted in his abdomen. (A Hospital C doctor had inserted the tube the day before the transfer, admitting afterward that he might have punctured Bill's colon in the process.)

Upon our arrival at Hospital D, our final hospital, every department head consulted on Bill's case during the first three hours—a far cry from the poorly coordinated reception he had received at the world-famous out-of-state facility. The surgeon came to me and said, "Your husband is about as sick as anyone can be and still be alive." His assistants scurried around, securing my permission to operate and advising me of the survival rate: less than 5 percent. At this point, we were so past probable survival I could barely digest the information. All I could do was get a room there for myself, pray, and try to rest up for the next day: in all probability, Bill's last day on this earth.

It was Saturday, not a day ordinarily chosen for surgery, but necessary for this time-critical procedure. Bill was somewhat alert that morning, so I told him what we were going to do: cut out the growths in his abdomen that were causing all the problems. I kissed him, silently praying it wasn't goodbye.

Then I joined the thirteen friends and family members who had miraculously showed up to provide support—miraculous in that they had flown from all over the country with less than twenty-four hours' notice, miraculous in that nurses who knew us "three hospitals ago" were present, miraculous in that they all loved both of us, even though the original friendships had begun with only one of us. We filled the waiting room, waiting to hear if the 5-percent survival rate had prevailed with my honey, my husband, my Bill. When the surgeon emerged following the surgery, his first response was, "Wow! What a crowd!"

As he assured us that Bill had done well throughout the surgery, a collective cry went up. He described removing four basketball-sized pseudocysts from Bill's abdomen, then packing it with surgical gauze to absorb the drainage and let the swelling go down. In two days he would go back to the surgical site to remove the gauze and close the wound. The surgeon sat with all of us patiently, answering questions for twenty minutes. We hail this man as the person who saved Bill's life.

Even though Bill went septic again that night and on many subsequent occasions at Hospital D, this surgery marked the turning point for his extraordinary recovery. Literally, from the moment he left surgery, Bill began to heal.

Several days after he finally regained consciousness, Bill began to write me notes. He was so weak that his letters were only about an eighth of an inch high, and they all ran together. The poor guy couldn't figure out why I couldn't read them! But he was now strong enough to ask the nurse to turn his bed around so he could see the helipad and watch the helicopters arrive with hospital patients.

He began physical and occupational therapy in earnest. I learned about and helped with his exercises and was the sole administrator of the same on weekends and holidays when the physical therapy (PT) and occupational therapy (OT) staff was not present.

I learned how to dress Bill's surgical sites and came to know the names and understand the purposes of the eleven drainage tubes and pumps implanted in his abdomen. I learned how to "deep suction" his trach and empty the traps of water collected in his ventilator tubing. By this time, he had developed MRSA: multi-resistant (or methicillin-resistant) staphylococcus aureus, also called a hospital-acquired infection or, in medical language, a "nosocomial" or "iatrogenic" infection. So now I had to wear a gown, mask, and gloves when in his room. I had also become quite handy at assisting with patient movement, foot massage, and boot replacement or removal. The boots are a device placed on the feet of long-term hospital patients to automatically squeeze and release the feet, thus preventing blood clots.

My skills and Bill's condition improved daily, so much so that by early March—five months after his initial hospital admission—he was strong enough to transfer out of Hospital D to the rehabilitation unit. Even his kidneys began working again and, although not perfect, they were functioning well enough that dialysis could be discontinued.

Always the optimist, I believed Bill's progress was now a certainty, although he still had occasional line infections and continual feeding tube problems. Slowly, doctors removed tubes and weaned him off the ventilator. He continued to improve. In late March, exhausted but comfortable with Bill's condition, I went to New Mexico for four days to relax—collapse was more like it.

On the Thursday after my trip, Bill complained to both me and the nurses about being quite tired. He was too tired to do his scheduled therapy that day and the next. Since this was not an uncommon complaint, neither the other healthcare providers nor I took it too seriously. On Friday, he complained of a headache and was quite crabby. For once I chose to go home that night to sleep in our bed because his behavior had worn me out.

At 6:30 the next morning, the phone beside my bed rang. I answered it and heard a nurse telling me to get to the hospital as fast as I could: Bill had coded in the rehab unit and been readmitted to intensive care. I threw on clothes and flew to the hospital. Once I got there, the doctor treating Bill told me that on a routine middle-of-the-night check, the care partner had come in to take his temperature and check his pulse, finding him barely breathing. She called a code, at which point he began having seizures and stopped breathing.

Because of the seizures, the doctors could barely get the ventilator tube down his throat—his trach opening had grown shut by then. His oxygen level registered at less than 60 percent, which could mean anywhere between 1 and 60: the equipment in use was not sensitive enough to measure below 60 percent. Because the medical team responding to the code could not get Bill's seizures under control, they artificially induced a coma. No one could give me a cause or a prognosis, physical or mental.

Bill was kept comatose and ventilated for six days while the doctors searched for a medication that would control his seizure activity. For some reason, his previously injured liver just ate up seizure medications, as it does to this day.

It took four tries, but finally Bill was finally "loaded" with a therapeutic level of Dilantin, the drug that had controlled his seizures the year before. He was weaned off his sedatives, and he returned to consciousness.

The next few weeks were ghastly, for Bill and all the rest of us. Bill continually reported he was in Chicago (we were in a different city). He wanted to go downtown and get some pizza (he was still NPO, which means "nothing by mouth"). He insisted on walking to the bathroom "like a man" (he couldn't even sit up unaided). He saw and heard a skinny little man under my bed who blew on an empty pop bottle during the night.

Behind this behavior was some new documented evidence: Bill's brain was damaged in the right frontal and temporal lobes. The damage was caused by suspected endocarditis, a heart-valve infection probably triggered by his MRSA. The infection had spread and seeded itself in multiple locations of his brain, causing more infection, seizures, and another stroke. It would be six to twelve months before we knew the true impact of this horrible episode, the doctors said. We would have to wait to see if his brain used its capability to regenerate new pathways.

I never dreamed I would get his body back for him, only to lose his mind.

Bill was confused; he periodically pulled out his tubes. Hospitals are *very* cautious about using restraints, but I approved the use of soft gloves without thumbs. Bill figured out how to get those off and soon was trying to get out of bed without help. I had to approve a more aggressive method of restraint: Bill's hands and feet were tied to the bed. Fortunately and surprisingly, his kidneys continued working throughout this trauma. His speech therapists, and his occupational and physical therapists, demonstrated great patience with his mentally limited repertoire. Slowly, slowly, Bill came around.

Due to his diligent progress, Hospital D discharged Bill on June 6, 2001, exactly seven and a half months after admission. In order to care for him at home, I learned how to administer IVs, give shots, dress wounds, and manage seizures at home. Bill still has a seizure disorder. When he has "break-through" seizures—particularly severe ones—he is treated by paramedics and at the hospital.

Today, more than six years later, Bill struggles with the reality of a changed life. The blessings are immense, and so are the losses. He had to wait for over a year and a half to drive—he had to stay seizure-free for six consecutive months before he was cleared to drive again. Then he had an accident in my car during an "absence seizure" when he was unaware of his surroundings: an episode caused by taking the generic equivalent of his seizure medication. Although no one was hurt, he had to wait another six months to drive again. He broke bones in his feet three times. The factors there were lack of weight-bearing activity and the onset of osteoporosis from six months of substandard feeding tube nutrition. Still, higher levels of nutrition might have placed too much stress on his newly recovered kidneys: in medicine, the tradeoffs can be complex.

Bill receives private disability and Social Security, something we never thought we would see in our lifetimes. Since leaving the hospital, Bill has done extensive physical therapy; he took up yoga for a time. He still tires easily. He continues to grapple with balance issues and has lost most of the sensation in his feet. His depression and anger can be overwhelming for both of us. But he is alive, and there is hope.

For patient advocates, there is a bottom line, and it is this: Never, never give up! There are miracles in the world. I know it, because Bill is one of them. Life is a gift: seek it.

# 14 KEY RECOMMENDATIONS

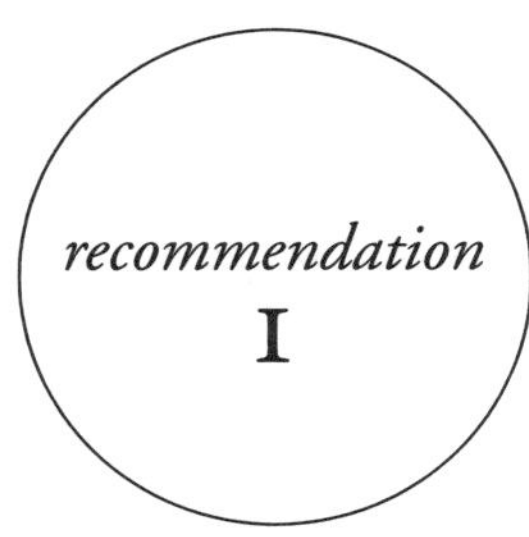
recommendation
I

# TAKE CARE *of Yourself*

You are of no value to your loved one if you go down for the count. Sacrificing your own health for another is not what anyone who loves you would want you to do.

*Fear is that little darkroom*
*where negatives are developed.*

—Michael Pritchard

Take good care of yourself: that is my first and last recommendation to you because all the others depend on it. Replenish yourself. What gives you strength or refreshes you when your energy is low? Remind yourself of those things, or seek answers now if you need to. This book is not meant to help you in that search; it is about caring for another who needs your help. But you cannot do this unless you care for yourself first.

I needed personal assistance, at various degrees at various times, in five areas: at home, at the hospital, physically, emotionally, and spiritually. Whichever area was "up" at a particular time, one key source of help was always available—my friends. But I had to learn to accept their help. I have always been very independent; generally I've been the one offering help to others. Accepting assistance was a foreign concept to me.

As a consultant working with employees in the "soft side" of business, behavioral change, I've often reminded myself that "People don't change unless the pain of remaining the same exceeds the pain of doing things differently." Well, during Bill's hospitalization, I finally applied that rule to myself. For me, the pain of remaining the same—stubbornly independent—was way more painful than accepting "a little help from my friends." Please let others "do" for you during this time.

## 1. At Home

If you stay with your loved one at the hospital, you will need help at home. If other people depend on you—children or elders—they will be your first concern. But many other tasks will need to be done, too. Find neighbors, family members, or friends to help with all of them.

Pets, for example. At the time of his illness, Bill and I had four dogs. We have always considered them part of our family, calling them our "kids." Several people offered to help (whether they liked dogs or not). But for the longer term, our former dog sitter, April, agreed to take care of them. I lent Bill's truck to April for that period of time, a trade that worked well for all of us.

If your home is empty, who will help you make it look occupied to prevent burglary? Who can lend a hand with maintenance? Since April was coming to the house three times a day, she also turned lights on and off at various times and left the truck sometimes in the driveway, sometimes in the garage, to create a natural inconsistency, should anyone be watching the house. Our housecleaner stayed on a regular schedule, checking in to make sure all was well and to handle any mishaps (such as the water pipes that froze during an unexpected cold snap). Other friends and neighbors picked up mail and newspapers.



One of the real joys in my life is my greenhouse. Bill had built it for me and customized it to meet my every desire. I have hundreds of plants, and my friend Kevin watered them weekly. April helped here, too, turning the greenhouse lights on and off and activating the heater, when needed.

When spring came and I could spare a little time away from the hospital to ready the house for Bill's homecoming, my sister's family and our friends spent many hours planting our annual garden, cleaning the gutters, and raking the leaves from the previous fall—all things that had gone undone during Bill's hospitalization.

Pets, houseplants, yard and garden, vehicles, home maintenance (including heat, power, and plumbing), vehicles, mail and packages, burglary prevention: think ahead and ask for help to cover all these areas.

## 2. At the Hospital

If you are essentially living at the hospital, you still need to eat and wear clean clothes. The hospital cafeteria may be a big help, especially if the food is both good and affordable, and the hours are generous. For me, meals at our first (underpopulated) hospital were a problem because the cafeteria only served breakfast and lunch—and only on weekdays. So friends brought me food galore. My sister did my laundry regularly and picked up my own medications from our pharmacy as needed. Life would have been difficult without everyone's help.

Consider your own physical comfort in the hospital room. In Hospital D, the chair bed in Bill's room was a real asset: a chair that I could convert into a bed by pulling out a section and rearranging the cushions. Even if you don't plan to sleep at the hospital, a chair bed can help you with an occasional catnap.

Find something to do in the hospital room. Even doing everything I could to help with Bill's care, I had huge amounts of time left over. Bring handwork, writing materials, any other projects that lend themselves to the setting. Bring reading material, and check the hospital library for magazines and books, which are available for checkout to family members. Walk the hospital and you'll find magazines in every waiting room. I borrowed these magazines freely, always returned them, and never heard a complaint. I also contributed to those reading stashes by adding my own magazines and catalogs. If you do this, however, remove your name and address from the mailing label and any inside order form before donating it to the cause. Let's not make life any easier for the identity thieves!

Protect your credit card number in the hospital, too. Destroy any paperwork or receipt that includes it: ideally, take it home to shred. In Bill's room, I once threw a credit-card purchase receipt into the in-room bag designated for contaminated substances. Big mistake. A thief found it and used it to buy a $3,000 computer online. And to find that receipt, the thief risked exposure to the bag's contents—blood, feces, and other body fluids, possibly carrying infectious disease—on the off chance of finding something of value. Fortunately, I caught the fraudulent charge early and my credit card company removed it from my bill.

Guard your physical security, too. Stay alert when entering or exiting the hospital, especially at night. Ask a security guard to accompany you to your car—you are particularly vulnerable if you are preoccupied, grieving, or in any way inattentive. Even in a patient room, be aware of people's presence—especially in hospitals with open-door visiting policies. Carry any valuable items with you at all times: purse or briefcase, electronic devices, and so on. Patient room thefts were reported to me in two hospitals.

### 3. Physically

Pay attention to your own physical health, lest you become a patient yourself. Watch for signs of stress in your body and do what you can to dissipate it. We all carry tension in particular places, often in areas that have been injured in the

past. My neck, previously injured in an auto accident, was so tight that on some days I couldn't turn my head. I asked friends for a referral to a massage therapist, and I'm glad I did. Exercise helps, too. If the hospital has a fitness center, ask if you can have a temporary membership.

Wash your hands often! This simple precaution helps protect both you and your loved one from contagion. Many hospital-acquired infections, such as MRSA, can be avoided by careful hand washing and other protocols to promote a sterile environment. If your clothing has come in contact with a patient with an infection, change out of it and launder it: neckties can easily carry infections this way. Consider removing and sanitizing your shoes when you're home after a hospital visit, especially if anyone in the household has a compromised immune system. Your purse or briefcase can also be a carrier of E. coli, so sanitize it weekly.

Drink lots of water. Hospitals are notoriously dry, and lack of water can take a big toll when coupled with stress. Give your body the water it needs. Find the water cooler on each floor and use it. I never realized how little water I drank until I saw how the staff measured and recorded every milliliter of liquid Bill took in. Some people find they can't wear contact lenses because of the dry hospital air. Friends brought me hand lotion and lip balm for the same reason.

Ground yourself. At least once a day, step outside, pause, take a walk, and orient yourself to the world outside your microcosm. It will provide perspective, oxygen, and a reality check. A friend taught me a simple exercise for these times: Take a deep breath and as you slowly exhale, visualize pushing all your tension into the ground. Repeat two more times. I found this ritual to be invaluable.

In fact, my own self-grounding was crucial not only to my health, but to Bill's survival. By grounding, I was able to stay calmer and less emotional (though certainly not unemotional!). And the calmer I was while talking with healthcare providers, the more receptive they were to me, and the more productive our conversation.

Notice, too, whether you are restless or irritable at certain times of day. ICU staff often see a pattern in certain patients that they call "sundowner's syndrome." Sundowning is a "state of increased agitation, activity and negative behaviors that happen late in the day through the evening hours,"[1] typically triggered by fatigue. Patients do get tired, even with very little activity. Bill suffered from sundowning on several occasions and still does, to some extent, at home when he is overtired. Guess who else was susceptible to sundowning? I was, and you will be, too, if you allow your 24/7 duty to keep you from leaving your loved one's side. Believe me, you actually do get tired sitting in a hospital room, if only from the anxiety!



### 4. Emotionally

A trusted medical adviser can be a big asset for you emotionally—an ally who is not directly involved in your loved one's care. I am not a trained medical professional; even when certified as an emergency medical technician (EMT) early in my career, I didn't have occasion to use those skills. But even had I been trained I would have needed help: Bill's case was too complex for any one healthcare professional to untangle alone. Sometimes doctors didn't fully agree with each other. Often a doctor described to me the pros and cons of a given course of action, then looked to me for a decision when Bill was incapacitated. As his spouse and advocate, it was up to me. I needed a trusted medical adviser to help me think through problems and make good choices.

I was lucky to have two medical advisers: our family physician and a friend who is a nurse practitioner. I discussed every incident with these two special and ever-patient partners. The physician also helped me cope with my anxiety. Without the help of these two allies, I would not have felt as confident about my decisions and probably would have second-guessed myself—especially if Bill had died. Not that the specialists treating Bill were incompetent and unhelpful—after all, they kept him viable through multiple catastrophic medical events! However, they were very clear about the limits of their abilities, and the choices they could not make. They provided me with excellent options. However, options in the plural required decisions in the singular—decisions only I could make. Without my outside medical advisers, I would have been lost.

---

1 Edyth Ann Knox, "Tips on . . . Sundowning," Eldercare online, http://www.ec-online.net/Knowledge/Articles/sundowntip.html.

We can only run on our emotional reserves for so long. We need others to help us replenish them. At the beginning, it was terrifying and nerve-racking not to know what caused Bill's illness. But we had reason for optimism: the doctors were anticipating "the normal run for pancreatitis," meaning seven to ten days in the hospital. At that time, there were lots of folks around to help, but I didn't open myself up to them. I was still running on my own reserves. But when the catastrophes commenced and continued, I went to my emotional well so many times that it dried up and collapsed into itself. That was when I learned to accept emotional support, a hard lesson for me. I learned to lean on others and let them share their strength, too.



"Lean number 1" occurred during Bill's first septic episode. Both my sister and Skip were by my side that night, literally telling me what to do, as I was numb and terrified. "Jari, why don't you take a walk and try to relax?" they asked. I didn't want to leave the bedside that night, but the point was well taken. After that, not only did I accept a strong shoulder, I even occasionally sought one out. When I flew Bill to the out-of-state hospital, I racked up $500 in cell phone charges, calling people just to talk, to lean on. By the time Bill went in for his surgery, thirteen friends, colleagues, and family members had arranged to be there, some coming from afar. This was a tremendous help, for had the outcome been different, I would have needed to lean on every one of them.

Throughout Bill's illness, unsolicited kindness and compassion came my way. This was good, because I hardly knew how to ask for it. Even if I hadn't been so needy, the sheer volume of love eventually would have gotten through. I only wish I had been able to accept it from the beginning. The Pueblo Indians speak the truth when they say, "The step beyond surrender is often magic."

## 5. Spiritually

The seriousness of a life-threatening illness will test and confirm your spiritual belief, even if you have to pull it out and dust it off from years of disuse.

Regardless of the nature of your spiritual belief, finding the chapel in the hospital should be one of the first things you do. Whether you define "God" according to Christianity, Judaism, or spiritualism, whether you have any kind of faith in a Higher Power greater than yourself or simply need some peace and quiet, the chapel offers solace at whatever level you desire.



In not one of the four hospitals did a chaplain ever enter the chapel while I sat in there. For me, that was a relief, as I went to the chapel for solitude. Just sitting quietly helped me with perspective and gave me relief from the noise of the machines keeping my husband alive. The chaplain did visit Bill's hospital room in each hospital, asking whether spiritual support was desired. That is the best time to work out the level of support both you and your loved one seek.

The question "Why me?" troubled me especially one day as I was communing with my Higher Power. I was reminded of a lesson I learned shortly after beginning my consulting business in 1986. For six months I helped a company set up its human resources function. As part of this project, I created its first-ever employee handbook, which contained, among its health-related matters, an AIDS policy. Acquired immune deficiency syndrome was, at that time, viewed as very different from other terminal or disabling diseases. Thus, the need for a separate policy.

There were some difficulties with this assignment so, as I do with all completed assignments, I turned around and looked back at it, conducting what I call an "autopsy of events." I do this so I can see what I learned or what I was supposed to learn. Try as I might, I could not find any significant learning for myself on this assignment. Troubled but not overly so, I moved on to my next assignment and gave it no more thought.

Two months later, at the request of a colleague at that company, I called one of the company officers, using the unfamiliar phone number he gave me. The officer answered and told me he was in the hospital and wanted me to visit. The evening I visited him, he disclosed that he had contracted AIDS and was in the final stage of the disease, with little time left.

We cried together, and he hugged me when I left, thanking me for implementing his company's AIDS policy so he could die in peace, knowing he and his family would not suffer financially. I left the hospital, shaken to the core. Not only was this the first person I had known who contracted AIDS, this was someone who attributed his peaceful departure to me.

For many days, I grappled with the sorrow of his impending death, and then I realized he had given me an enormous gift. That assignment had finally given me a lesson: a lesson in humility and responsibility. In this case, I was just the servant who did my job. In doing so, I stumbled upon the right thing to do, convinced the company it was so, and set in motion a chain of events that neither I nor the employer could have expected.



I tell this story to remind you that the hospitalization of your loved one is not about you! You may be an innocent bystander. But remember, bystanders save strangers' lives every day, and your family member is hardly a stranger. Do what you can. In the process, you, too, may receive an enormous gift, the gift of life.

Spirituality also came to me through the other people trying to cope with Bill's illness. Each of us seeks spirit in our own way; who's to say which is the right way? I honor all the prayers said for Bill and me, whether spoken in English or not, whether said in a church or a synagogue or in bed at night, whether spoken by a Muslim or a Catholic. My "God" heard and answered them all. Nikos Kazantzakis tells us this about God: "God changes appearances every second. Blessed is the man who can recognize him in all his disguises. One moment he is a glass of fresh water, the next, your son bouncing on your knees or an enchanting woman, or perhaps merely a morning walk."[2]

**Checklist A**, which follows, reflects these five areas of self-care: at home, at the hospital, physically, emotionally, and spritually. Use it, and add items to it, to help yourself stay organized and to promote your own peace of mind.

2 Nikos Kazantzakis, *Zorba the Greek* (New York: Scribner Paperback Fiction, 1981).

1

Take Care of Yourself

## *Checklist A: Taking Care of Me*

| CATEGORY | ARRANGEMENTS NEEDED | ✓ |
|---|---|---|
| At home | Child care | |
| | Elder care | |
| | Pet care | |
| | Plants, yard, garden | |
| | Lights for security | |
| | Home maintenance | |
| | Mail | |
| | Vehicles | |
| | | |
| | | |
| At the hospital | Round-the-clock patient coverage | |
| | Food | |
| | Sleeping arrangements | |
| | Personal items (purse, briefcase, tote) | |
| | Electronic devices as allowed by hospital | |
| | Journal, paper and tape to make and post signs | |
| | Reading material, handwork, and so on | |
| | | |
| | | |
| Physically | Walking and other exercise | |
| | Stress relief | |
| | Grounding: calming and centering techniques | |
| | Frequent hand washing | |
| | Sanitization of shoes, clothing, personal items | |
| | Drinking adequate water | |
| | Medications | |
| | | |
| | | |

*Checklist A (continued)*

| CATEGORY | ARRANGEMENTS NEEDED | ✓ |
|---|---|---|
| Emotionally | Family phone numbers | |
| | Friends' phone numbers | |
| | Trusted medical advisor[s] phone number[s] | |
| | | |
| | | |
| | | |
| Spiritually | Location of hospital chapel | |
| | Spiritual advisor[s] phone number | |
| | Ways to notify patient's faith community | |
| | | |
| | | |
| | | |

recommendation
2

# CHOOSE YOUR HOSPITAL *with Awareness*

HOSPITALS WITH FEWER patients generally offer more thorough nursing care but less doctor presence. Overpopulated hospitals offer more doctor availability—but at the expense of care. If you have to choose, which is more important for your loved one: nursing care or doctor presence?

*He who asks a question is a fool for five minutes;*
*he who does not ask a question remains a fool forever.*
—CHINESE PROVERB

Aren't all hospitals more or less the same? some of us might wonder. The answer to that question is no, but the extent of their differences may surprise you. It surprised me. I'm a business consultant who knows very well that every company and institution is unique. But until Bill's illness I had never considered hospitals in that light.

Over seven months, Bill was a patient in four hospitals: two were intentionally chosen, two were accidental. During that time, I learned a great deal about the differences between hospitals. Every one has strengths and weaknesses. Naturally, so do doctors. You may have a choice to make there, too. So if you are planning a stay, practice due diligence—in other words, do your homework. Your reward will be a facility with the best combination of factors to support your patient's recovery.

## Some General Strategies

First, consider which hospitals are available to you as an "in-plan" option through your insurance carrier—that may rule some out right away. Then, do your homework. If you have time before the hospitalization, discuss with your loved one what will matter most about their support and recovery. Your preferred physician may practice at a certain hospital, but that doesn't necessarily make that hospital the ideal choice for your situation. It may simply be a hospital in which the doctor has a financial interest. Given time, there are always options. Learn all you can about what the patient will need, and look for that. It might be that excellent nursing care is more crucial to your loved one's recovery than the presence of a particular doctor.

The one must-have for your hospital is accreditation by the Joint Commission, formerly known as the Joint Commission on Accreditation of Healthcare Organizations (JCAHO). This group inspects and certifies healthcare facilities against predetermined standards. Call 630-792-5000 for general information, or visit www.jointcommission.org. To review its most up-to-date accreditation results, visit www.qualitycheck.org/consumer/searchQCR/aspx.

There is no perfect formula for a "best hospital," as every situation is different. It is often, to some extent, a balancing act: Which pros and cons are most important in your patient's case? What are the tradeoffs?

## Case Study: Comparing Four Hospitals

As an example, let's look at the four hospitals in which Bill was treated, as seen through my eyes—their general strengths and weaknesses. Then we'll compare them item for item: a process that may help you decide the features to look for, and the questions to ask, as you choose your own hospital.



### *Hospital A: Private facility*

Hospital A happened to be near Bill's workplace, and he was transported there in emergency mode. So we did not choose it ahead of time, but we found it satisfactory. At this hospital Bill was treated by what I came to call his primary doctors—a GI, or gastrointestinal ("gut") specialist, a nephrologist (kidney specialist), and a pulmonologist (respiratory or lung specialist). He spent seven weeks here on full life support, much of that time in a coma. He had his tracheotomy, experienced his first septic episodes, and developed pseudocysts. Medically, he was a very challenging patient.

The single biggest advantage of Hospital A was its low patient count. It is unusual for any medical facility to have a one-to-one nurse-to-patient ratio, even in the intensive care unit, where Bill was throughout his stay. But here it happened that Bill had a nurse assigned only to him. With no competing priorities, that nurse's attention was fully focused where it was needed or requested.

In this case, Bill did the needing and I did the requesting. My requests had to do with helping me understand Bill's treatments, equipment, and generally what was going on. Once my initial panic had passed, I began asking questions about everything, and Bill's nurses were generous with their time, knowledge, and compassion. I learned more here than at the next three hospitals combined.

We were privileged to have two of the hospital's best and most seasoned nurses included in the shift rotation. And thanks to its "continuity of care," Bill repeatedly was cared for by the same nurses—a significant advantage for any patient, but particularly for one with such complex and ever-changing conditions. Here Bill survived catastrophic medical events directly as a result of this attentive nursing care.

This hospital's single biggest disadvantage, however, was also its low patient count: this asset also has a flip side. With so few patients, the doctor presence was low, and MDs were rarely present during Bill's continuing crises. His primary team generally made daily rounds on weekdays—although even that was minimal attention, considering his deterioration and the complexity of his illness. And on night, weekend, and holiday shifts, typically there was only one doctor on duty in the entire hospital. The only way to get that doctor into Bill's room was for him to "code"—that is, to have a life-threatening episode, also called "code blue" in medical jargon. So during these shifts, the doctor on duty never had time to focus on ongoing and preventive care—Bill became a priority only during and after a crisis.

### *Hospital B: World-renowned teaching/research facility*

This hospital was recommended for its extensive experience in treating Bill's illness. This time, we had a choice, and I chose this facility over Hospital D based on my knowledge of its international reputation. We would soon learn that reputation can be misleading.

Bill was airlifted to Hospital B's ICU, then spent ten days under the care of doctors who rejected his earlier diagnosis until they could confirm it for themselves. Their prognosis was grim going in, and it stayed that way. Meanwhile, Bill was denied dialysis, leading to a dangerous cardioversion episode. He was also denied a rotating bed, which led to bedsores. There was no continuity of nursing care, despite repeated requests: new nurses were constantly having to learn about his condition and his needs. He was assigned a "gatekeeper" doctor to coordinate care. In Bill's case this complicated matters because the gatekeeper had to approve all treatments in advance.

We had such a bad experience here, I have trouble identifying anything positive. But even if his care had been outstanding technically, the manner in which we were treated would still have made it a miserable experience. Frankly, the air of superiority that pervaded Hospital B colored our every interaction with staff. They seemed to look down on us—not an attitude that promotes healing. On all levels, this facility was a huge disappointment.

### *Hospital C: Another private facility*

Bill was transported directly from Hospital B to Hospital C. I had been given a choice between trying this hospital and returning to our first facility. I chose Hospital C in consult with Bill's nephrologist, who practiced there. That, coupled with the need for more onsite doctor availability than Hospital A, made the choice a clear one. By selecting this facility, Bill was again treated by his original team of three primary doctors.

Bill was still on full life support at Hospital C. Now intermittently awake, he was still in intensive care, with ascites enlarging his absomen. His care was satisfactory, but his stay was short here, too: just ten days.

### *Hospital D: University teaching facility*

I chose this facility when Bill's pancreatic pseudocysts became infected and surgery was mandatory. I was now given the choice of Hospital B or D. Since we had already been there and done that—miserably—with Hospital B, there really was no alternative.

We were at Hospital D for the longest period: five months. We experienced all levels of care here, whereas our stays up to this point had been in intensive care only. And here he had the surgery that saved his life.

At this point in Bill's disease, doctor expertise would make the difference between life and death. The doctors in Hospital D were very seasoned. At this facility, research is expected and rewarded, and the doctors applied cutting-edge techniques in the treatment of many of Bill's conditions. The surgeon obviously was excellent. But once again, the flip side of this advantage meant a disadvantage.

The doctors here were what I call "body part specialists": all were highly skilled experts, but focused on only one part of the body. And there was no staff hospitalist serving as "general contractor" to oversee the whole patient. Although there were care coordinators who played a similar role, I found myself acting as the glue to keep Bill's treatments and procedures coordinated. This was three months into his illness: I was no rookie, and I felt comfortable with my role. But for a new advocate, it could be a lot to handle.

Another minor tradeoff: in this teaching hospital, Bill was often the "lesson of the day" for medical students, entailing repeated conversations with physicians in various specialities and stages of training. Moreover, because Hospital D accepted uninsured patients, it meant that even insured patients sometimes had to wait for admission, treatment, transfer, and discharge. Nonetheless, this facility and its expertise saved Bill's life, for which I will forever be grateful.

### *Four hospitals: Surveying strengths and weaknesses*

The chart on the next two pages shows my ratings, in retrospect, of each hospital's performance on a number of criteria. The column on the left lists features that are generally desirable; the ratings are on a four-point scale where 1 = outstanding, 2 = good, 3 = neutral, and 4 = poor.

A note on the second feature listed: "Effective hospitalist or other staff coordinating 'whole-patient' care." Although the presence of a hospitalist speaks well for the facility, other staff can do the job, such as nurse care coordinators or nurse practitioners. The title is less important than the person's effectiveness. Here is some background on my ratings for that criterion: Hospital A = 1 (outstanding). The hospitalist's role was well integrated into the treatment protocol: ours was a visible team member who was generous with sharing time. Hospital B = 4 (poor). With no hospitalists here, the ICU head took that role—but served not so much as a coordinator as a gatekeeper who had to approve every treatment decision, often raising roadblocks. There was no partnering with the patient advocate. Hospital C = 3 (neutral). The facility did have staff hospitalists, but they were not visible, and their presence was of questionable significance. Hospital D = 2 (good). Although there were no hospitalists here, nurse care coordinators served this function well, partnering with the patient advocate.

### *Comparing Our Four Hospitals*

*This chart shows how each hospital rated on each of the preferred criteria listed at the left. 1 = outstanding, 2 = good, 3 = neutral, 4 = poor.*

| PREFERRED CONDITIONS | Hosp A | Hosp B | Hosp C | Hosp D |
|---|---|---|---|---|
| **General conditions of care** | | | | |
| General availability of health care providers | 1 | 3 | 3 | 2 |
| Effective hospitalist or other staff coordinating "whole-patient" care | 1 | 4 | 3 | 1 |
| General openness to family involvement in care; willingness to teach | 1 | 4 | 3 | 2 |
| General friendliness | 1 | 4 | 3 | 1 |
| Good protocols to prevent contagion | 4 | 1 | 2 | 1 |
| General affordability of care | 4 | 2 | 3 | 1 |
| **Doctors** | | | | |
| Favorable doctor-to-patient ratio | 4 | 3 | 2 | 1 |
| Doctor expertise in our particular medical needs | 4 | 2 | 3 | 1 |
| Doctors made rounds at fairly predictable times | 2 | 4 | 3 | 1 |
| Doctors made rounds together and/or consulted with each other reliably | 1 | 4 | 1 | 4 |
| Primary doctor's partners were of equally high quality | 4 | 2 | 4 | 1 |
| Weekday availability of backup doctors if needed | 4 | 2 | 2 | 1 |
| Night/weekend/holiday availability of backup doctors | 4 | 3 | 3 | 1 |
| **Nursing and other staff** | | | | |
| Favorable nurse-to-patient ratio | 1 | 4 | 2 | 4 |
| Highly skilled nursing care | 1 | 3 | 3 | 2 |
| Good consistency and continuity of nursing care | 1 | 4 | 2 | 1 |
| Quick responses from pharmacy and lab staff | 1 | 2 | 3 | 4 |
| Availability of chaplain | 1 | 4 | 4 | 2 |

*Continued on next page*

*Comparing Our Four Hospitals (continued)*

| PREFERRED CONDITIONS | Hosp A | Hosp B | Hosp C | Hosp D |
|---|---|---|---|---|
| **Facility and equipment** | | | | |
| Fairly new facility (fewer "resident germs" than in older facilities) | 1 | 4 | 2 | 4 |
| State-of-the-art equipment | 1 | 3 | 2 | 2 |
| Needed equipment available quickly | 1 | 4 | 2 | 2 |
| Needed supplies available quickly | 4 | 2 | 2 | 1 |
| Patient rooms of adequate size | 1 | 2 | 4 | 3 |
| Adequate linen service | 4 | 1 | 2 | 3 |
| **Visitor policies / amenities** | | | | |
| 24-hour visitor access (or only slight restrictions) | 1 | 4 | 4 | 2 |
| Family members often allowed in room during procedures | 1 | 4 | 4 | 2 |
| Sleeping accommodations provided for family (separate room or in-room) | 1 | 4 | 4 | 3 |
| Digital cell phones permitted (if not interfering with medical equipment) | 1 | 4 | 3 | 2 |
| Cafeteria: quality, variety, affordability; generous hours | 4 | 1 | 1 | 4 |
| **Other access issues** | | | | |
| Easy access to patient's medical records (for family members) | 1 | 4 | 3 | 2 |
| Easy access to hospital management and administration | 1 | 4 | 4 | 2 |
| Easy access to medical library and/or resources | 4 | 1 | 2 | 4 |
| Good quality, up-to-date medical library / resources | 4 | 1 | 2 | 4 |
| Easy access to support groups and/or networks | 1 | 4 | 2 | 2 |

## Evaluate the Hospitals You're Considering

Those 1-to-4 ratings are, of course, an after-the-fact evaluation. If you're choosing your hospital, you'll be gathering information in advance and, where necessary, making educated guesses about how a given hospital will rate. To be realistic, I suggest you simply try to determine whether a given feature seems to be an area of strength or weakness. To do this, use **Checklist D: Hospital Evaluation** on pages 43–45: make a separate copy for each hospital you're considering. Listed on the left are all the features of the previous chart: add more as you see fit. The other columns are for your evaluations—does this seem to be strength or a weakness?—and your comments.



First, take these three steps as you screen hospitals for further evaluation: (1) Find out if it is included in your insurance policy's in-plan network. (2) Consider location: How convenient is it for you (and others) to spend a lot of time there? And can you get help managing the home front if needed? (3) If possible, discuss priorities with your loved one. Is your number one choice of doctor of primary importance? If you have to choose between that number one doctor and highly skilled nursing care, which would you value more? And ask open-ended questions to help your loved one "think out loud" about these priorities.

To prepare to fill out the Hospital Evaluation, you'll need to gather information, too. Use **Checklists B and C** for that.

### *Gathering information from doctor and hospital*

How can you be sure about a hospital's quality of care until you actually experience it? To be frank, you cannot. But for information and insight, ask questions of both the doctor and the hospital.

In many cases, doctors recommend the hospital where they themselves have privileges: that is, they are authorized to practice medicine there. That may be a good choice, but don't assume so. **Checklist B,** on page 40, shows some questions to ask your doctor about that facility, and about his or her experience. As you talk, notice the quality of your interaction, too, especially your doctor's listening abilities.

Then gather some information from the hospital staff: see **Checklist C** on pages 41–42. But where do you start? Think twice before going to staff in the general administration, patient advocacy, or public relations departments. They may be fine for certain standard facts. But you may not always get good, balanced information here: these staff will tend to "spin" their answers to promote the hospital. You may end up talking with the staff "patient advocate," too, but look elsewhere first—that person is in fact paid by the hospital, creating the potential for a conflict of interest. And admissions staff can discuss only the business aspects of a patient's stay.

What are better sources? I found that nurse specialists, also known as care coordinators, were reliable straight-shooters. Another valuable source are the doctors known as "hospitalists"—if the hospital has such MDs on staff. In fact, the presence of a hospitalist or a care coordinator is a big plus—an important factor in hospital choice, especially if the patient has a fairly complex health problem.

Hospitalists and care coordinators are the answer to these questions: with multiple specialists often caring for the same patient, who keeps the big picture in mind? Who coordinates that care?[1] The hospitalist serves as a "general contractor of healthcare," making sure the specialists are working in tandem, not at cross-purposes, that continuity of care is seamless, and that nothing is overlooked or confused for lack of a unified view of the patient. The hospitalist is a particular type of specialist—a very knowledgeable generalist—and it's the fastest-growing role in medicine.[2] The hospitalist also oversees the "hand-off" of the patient from the primary care physician at the beginning of the stay, and back again afterward.

In the words of one expert, "The hospitalist field was founded on the premise that inpatient generalists could improve the care of hospitalized patients and systems of inpatient care . . . In addition to their clinical work, hospitalists have

---

1 In a survey published in 2005, 43 percent of U.S. respondents reported problems when four doctors were providing care to one patient—by far the highest percentage of the six countries surveyed. Commonwealth Fund International Health Policy Survey, "Health System Views and Experiences Among Sicker Adults in Six Countries," *Health Affairs*, http://content.healthaffairs.org/content/vol0/issue2005/images/data/hlthaff.w5.509/DC1/Schoen_Nov_Ex5.gif.

2 Robert M. Wachter, "The Hospitalist Movement 10 Years Later: Life as a Swiss Army Knife," *Medscape General Medicine* 8, no. 3 (Aug. 4, 2006), http://www.medscape.com/viewarticle/540918.

become key leaders in quality, patient safety, information technology, palliative care, medical education, and more . . . In both settings, surgeons are clamoring for hospitalists to help 'co-manage' their patients."[3]

Indeed, doctors are even more pressed for time today than in years past, when the average full-time primary care physician might see only ten to twelve patients daily in the hospital. Today they see far more patients, and they may not be reimbursed for those visits, either. (They may also be very busy in their own offices, too, as more procedures are done on an in-office or outpatient basis.) Doctors must also keep abreast of the developments in their field, which may affect their recommendations for a given patient. All these issues point to the need for the hospitalist role.[4]



If a hospital has no care coordinators or hospitalists on staff, the patient advocate may be your best bet, and after all, you may ultimately need that person's help. Whoever you speak to, don't be afraid to bring your checklist with you. Introduce yourself, explain the purpose of your visit, and move into your questions. Take notes in the "Comments" column. Remember, the people with whom you are meeting are employees of the hospital and expected to support it. Listen carefully to what they say—and what they do not say.

For extra insight, consider stopping by a few hospital units, briefly walking around and paying attention to what you see and hear. Find out where the risk management office is and ask about their infection control procedures. (This is unusual for a family member to do, so you may meet with some resistance. But stiff resistance may suggest a general attitude of unwillingness to partner with you—a possible red flag.)

You might drop by the hospital cafeteria, too, and casually listen to the conversations around you. It is amazing what you can learn from unofficial sources!

---

3 Ibid.

4 James J. Foody, "The Hospitalist Movement 2003" from *Medscape Internal Medicine*, June 3, 2003, http://www.medscape.com/viewarticle/455915.

*Checklist B: Gathering Information from/about Your Doctor*

| QUESTIONS FOR THE DOCTOR | COMMENTS |
|---|---|
| With which hospital are you affiliated? Why? | |
| If multiple hospitals were available, which would you choose under these circumstances? | |
| What circumstances are driving your recommendation? | |
| What are the drawbacks of the recommended hospital? | |
| Tell me about the other doctors you would be consulting or working with to provide treatment. | |
| If my questions need more discussion time than you have, who will you make available to me—and why this person? | |
| How many cases like this have you treated in the last year? | |
| What kind of follow-up contact can we expect from you? | |
| What contact, if any, will we have with your partners? | |
| If appropriate, will I be allowed in the room during the procedure? | |
| Tell me about the quality of nursing care at the recommended hospital. | |
| Do you have a financial interest in this institution? | |

### *Checklist C: Gathering Information about Your Hospital*

| QUESTIONS FOR HOSPITAL STAFF | COMMENTS |
|---|---|
| Is this facility accredited by the Joint Commission (formerly known as JCAHO)? When was your last inspection? (Verify this with the Joint Commission.) | |
| What are your visiting policies? | |
| Will I be allowed to assist with the care of my family member? | |
| What kind of continuity of nursing care can I expect? | |
| What kind of spiritual support does this facility provide? | |
| Tell me about staffing levels for doctors and nurses on night shifts, weekends, and holidays. How do they compare with weekday shifts? | |
| May I look at a typical patient room? | |
| How old is this facility? When did you last remodel? | |
| What is the ratio of *registered* nurses (RNs) to patients in the specific service where my family member will be housed? (Specify RNs, as the nursing staff includes other personnel.) | |
| Tell me about (show me) your library. | |

*Continued on next page*

*Checklist C (continued)*

| QUESTIONS FOR HOSPITAL STAFF | COMMENTS |
|---|---|
| Tell me about your cafeteria. (Eat there and check it out for yourself.) | |
| Will I be allowed to see the labs and test results myself? | |
| May I use my digital cell phone on the premises? | |
| Describe your infection control procedures. | |
| What is the hospital's IV line change-out frequency? | |
| If I plan on sleeping at the hospital, do you have chair beds or rollaway beds or must I provide my own? | |
| Who will be the "general contractor" of my family member's healthcare—do you have hospitalists or care coordinators on staff? | |
| What is the protocol if I am dissatisfied with the care my family member is receiving? | |
| Do you use a computerized prescription/ records system? Do you keep backup hard copies of these records? How accessible are they? What happens when the computer goes down? | |

## *Checklist D: Hospital Evaluation*

*Make a copy of this three-page checklist for each hospital you are considering. Does each feature seem to be a strength or a weakness?*

| PREFERRED CONDITIONS | STRENGTH ✓ | WEAKNESS ✓ | COMMENTS |
|---|---|---|---|
| **General conditions of care** | | | |
| General availability of health care providers | | | |
| Effective hospitalist or other staff coordinating "whole-patient" care | | | |
| General openness to family involvement in care; willingness to teach | | | |
| General friendliness | | | |
| Good protocols to prevent contagion | | | |
| General affordability of care | | | |
| **Doctors** | | | |
| Favorable doctor-to-patient ratio | | | |
| Doctor expertise in our particular medical needs | | | |
| Doctors make rounds at fairly predictable times | | | |
| Doctors make rounds together and/or consult with each other reliably | | | |
| Primary doctor's partners are of equally high quality | | | |
| Weekday availability of backup doctors if needed | | | |
| Night/weekend/holiday availability of backup doctors | | | |

*Continued on next page*

*Checklist D (continued)*

| PREFERRED CONDITIONS | STRENGTH ✓ | WEAKNESS ✓ | COMMENTS |
|---|---|---|---|
| **Nursing and other staff** | | | |
| Favorable nurse-to-patient ratio | | | |
| Highly skilled nursing care | | | |
| Good consistency and continuity of nursing care | | | |
| Quick responses from pharmacy and lab staff | | | |
| Availability of chaplain | | | |
| **Facility and equipment** | | | |
| Fairly new facility (fewer "resident germs" than in older facilities) | | | |
| State-of-the-art equipment | | | |
| Needed equipment available quickly | | | |
| Needed supplies available quickly | | | |
| Patient rooms of adequate size | | | |
| Adequate linen service | | | |
| **Visitor policies / amenities** | | | |
| 24-hour visitor access (or only slight restrictions) | | | |
| Family members often allowed in room during procedures | | | |

*Checklist D (continued)*

| PREFERRED CONDITIONS | STRENGTH ✓ | WEAKNESS ✓ | COMMENTS |
|---|---|---|---|
| Sleeping accommodations provided for family (separate room or in-room) | | | |
| Digital cell phones permitted (if not interfering with medical equipment) | | | |
| Cafeteria: quality, variety, affordability; generous hours | | | |
| **Other access issues** | | | |
| Easy access to patient's medical records (for family members) | | | |
| Easy access to hospital management and administration | | | |
| Easy access to medical library and/or resources | | | |
| Good quality, up-to-date medical library / resources | | | |
| Easy access to support groups and/or networks | | | |

*recommendation*
3

# PICK THE DAYS OF YOUR STAY *Carefully*

Many hospitals go into a "holding pattern" for night shifts, weekends, and holidays. Few important procedures are done at those times, and staffing levels may be low.

*Holidays are an expensive trial of strength.*
*The only satisfaction comes from survival.*
—Jonathan Miller

3

*Pick the Days of Your Stay Carefully*

For optimal access to care, plan your hospital stay for a weekday period if possible, ideally with Monday admission. Even hospitals with an appropriate doctor presence may offer somewhat substandard care on night, weekend, and holiday shifts. Especially on holidays, the least experienced staff are often on duty because those with seniority bid for time off. And very few procedures are scheduled for those times. For Bill's entire hospitalization, only one crucial event ever took place on a weekend: his surgery. Had he not been so ill, it probably would have been postponed from Saturday to Monday, at which point it might well have cost him his life.

Nights, weekends, and holidays are also typically the time of lowest staffing (albeit with higher pay), adding to patients' vulnerability. Except in emergencies, it's in the patient's best interest not to be admitted just before a weekend or holiday, and it's preferable to be discharged by a Friday or by the eve of the holiday.

On Mother's Day during Bill's stay in Hospital D, one nurse handled an entire floor of sixteen patients for twelve hours, assisted by one care partner. When do you suppose that nurse got a break? Even with the best intentions, how clear-headed was she while distributing medications at 6 PM after ten hours? When one of her patients coded during the shift, she had to stay by his side and assist the emergency team for two hours until he was transferred to the intensive care unit. I wonder who was attending to the other fifteen patients? I know who was caring for my husband—I was. But what if another patient had needed immediate care?

Bill was in Hospital A's ICU on Thanksgiving Day. That night, Bill's triple lumen—a port that links three lines to one IV site—accidentally got caught in the rotating mattress and was pulled out.

This was no one's fault. However, it constituted an immediate need, as Bill was receiving both food and medications through this line. The ICU nurse first noticed it when she checked on Bill and saw one of the lines leaking all over the bed. A competent nurse, she had gained my respect by nursing Bill through the near-death experience of his second septic episode. She was, however, an agency nurse—not employed by the hospital, but subcontracted through an agency—and as such, she had to notify the nurse manager in charge before she made any requests. The nurse manager came to Bill's room, verified that the triple lumen was out, and said she would contact the hospitalist. I asked why, given that in three earlier instances an anesthesiologist had inserted the triple lumen. She answered that the hospital was short-staffed due to the holiday and proceeded to contact the hospitalist. When she reached him, I wasn't surprised that he recommended that an anesthesiologist replace the triple lumen. To her credit, she then contacted an anesthesiologist—who asked if the hospitalist could do the replacement. Clearly, she was getting the runaround.



At that point, the nurse manager made a decision with which I vehemently disagreed. Instead of insisting that the anesthesiologist come and do the job, she finished the call and told me, "It's a holiday and people are at home with their families, where they should be." When I asked if she was suggesting Bill couldn't get a medically necessary treatment because it was a holiday, she reiterated they were short-staffed and the triple lumen replacement could wait until the next morning.

By now, as a result of the missing line, Bill's blood pressure had risen. He had missed the bicarbonate that moderated the acid in his body, he had been without IV-administered food for over two hours, and he was about to miss his antibiotic treatment. Tired and frightened, I lost it. "No, it can't wait!" I told her. Was this really a twenty-four-hour ICU? I demanded she get help.

I had reason to question her judgment. Earlier I had seen her trying to pull nurses off Bill's care during an emergency, saying, "It only takes one person to care for him"—this during a septic episode with five nurses and a doctor barely keeping up with the required treatments. At other times, she had admonished me for washing my hands in the utility room when the sink in Bill's room was in use, and she had lectured me on changing my own sheets instead of "bothering" the housekeeping staff—lesser transgressions, but insensitive just the same.

So at my insistence, the nurse manager again called the hospitalist. While we waited for his return call, the agency nurse started an IV line. When she said we needed another line in addition to that one, I said no. By now I knew that for many reasons, it was hard to find a suitable site to "stick" Bill—hospital slang for inserting a needle. If the triple lumen was replaced, we could stop sticking him.

The hospital's pharmacy staff was available by pager. But rather than contacting them, the nurse manager called the pharmacies in two "sister" hospitals asking if there was an alternative delivery method for the antibiotic—asking the question within my earshot and without a full explanation of the situation. Neither pharmacist was aware of any other delivery method.

An hour and a half went by. When the anesthesiologist and hospitalist both arrived at the same time (the anesthesiologist because she had been requested, the hospitalist because he was worried), the triple lumen was replaced. When the hospitalist asked the nurse manager why Bill's primary doctor had not been called, she told him, "I'm not waiting around here anymore. I'm going home to be with my family. Here's my home phone number. He can call me there if he wants."

This episode brought me to the hospital's administrative offices the next day, where I reported it and requested that the nurse manager be banned from treating Bill or consulting in any way on his case. This request was honored for the rest of his stay. I later learned that the nurse manager had been suspended for her actions that night and was eventually terminated.

Although not typical, this incident shows the potential for problems during holiday shifts. The same holds true for nights and weekends. One Saturday midnight at Hospital D, after a nurse had been informed four times that one of Bill's medications was unavailable until Monday, I called the pharmacy manager at home myself. The nursing staff listened to my end of the call and indicated their support for my complaint. They later told me that "this happens all the time" but, as hospital employees, they were afraid to report it! They feared undermining their working relationship with the pharmacist—a fear that, itself, was undermining their patients' best interests.

If the staff is considering discharging your loved one on a Monday, ask what treatments they have planned for the weekend. If they say they simply want to watch the patient, ask if you can't do the same at home.

Although the night, weekend, and holiday syndrome is best avoided, one time it actually worked in our favor. On that same Mother's Day at Hospital D, the nurse in charge let me bring our Rhodesian Ridgeback dog into Bill's hospital room "through the back door." Obviously, family pets are not typically allowed. The hospital did have a pet therapy program at that time—a wonderful thing—but because Bill was MRSA positive, the program staff wasn't allowed into his room. Bill hadn't seen his own four-legged family members for more than six months, and this clandestine canine visit truly helped his mood. Precisely because of the absence of staff on the holiday, this nurse felt freer to bend the rules.

I would have traded this visit in a heartbeat, however, for more consistently competent care during the many nights, weekends, and holidays we spent in four hospitals. So be aware of this syndrome, and don't let these often substandard shifts cost you the life of your loved one. Maintain extra vigilance—and if anyone questions your attitude, you might answer, "I'm not tense, just terribly, terribly alert."

*recommendation*
4

# TAKE LEGAL STEPS TO *Ensure the Patient's Wishes Are Honored*

REQUEST THAT YOUR loved one prepare a living will and grant a chosen person Durable Medical Power of Attorney, preferably before entering the hospital. If needed later, these documents will help guide healthcare decisions. Other legal documents may also merit review.

*It's been emphatically proven that even seeds that appear dead—that is to say, were incapable of bearing life—for thousands of years, because of the conditions in which they were kept, can, given the appropriate conditions, suddenly bloom.*

—VANESSA REDGRAVE

4

*Take Legal Steps to Ensure the Patient's Wishes Are Honored*

Talk about a case of the cobbler's children not having shoes! I was married to an attorney who refused to deal personally with end-of-life legal issues such as a living will and durable medical power of attorney: it was "too upsetting to think about them." Therefore, Bill entered the hospital with no such documents on file. And I entered this medical nightmare as "just a spouse," not as a person legally authorized to make healthcare decisions on Bill's behalf. There is a big difference! Our lives were greatly simplified when I obtained a durable medical power of attorney document.

Also vitally important is a living will, which specifies a person's medical wishes if unable to make decisions at a later date. In some states, these two documents (and possibly others) are combined into one document, often called an advance directive. Ideally, these legal steps are taken *before* a hospital stay, but they may be done at any time.

Because this is such a personal matter, the advice below is addressed directly to the patient. It also assumes that the advance directive is the norm in your state, but state laws vary, so consult your hospital for your state's specifics. (See also the sample forms in appendix A.) Also included here as a "case study" is the story of my experience with and without a durable medical power of attorney document during Bill's illness.

Please read this recommendation carefully and share it with your patient as needed.

## The Advance Directive: Some Advice Straight to the Patient

Why do you need an advance directive? As a patient, you will have to make decisions about your medical care. But what if you are unconscious, unable to speak, or in a coma? If you have not previously shared your care wishes with family or friends, the medical community will make those decisions for you. (Recall the Terri Schiavo case that made headlines in 2005: the whole nation saw how one family was torn by the absence of an advance directive.)

The advance directive protects your rights as a patient. It is a legal document that allows you to designate a person to speak for you if you are unable to communicate. It also lets you specify your wishes for the types and extent of medical

treatment you wish to have—or not have—under certain circumstances. When an advance directive is in place, a note is placed in your medical file so all providers know of its existence. Be reassured: it will be used to govern healthcare decisions *only* if you are no longer able to communicate your wishes to the medical providers.

Federal law protects your right to choose whether to execute an advance directive or not: you are not required to in order to receive medical care. If you do execute one, your hospital may not use it to condition your care or discriminate against you; it must continue to provide quality medical care. Your healthcare team has the same duty.

The key documents included in an advance directive are (1) the Durable Medical Power of Attorney and (2) the living will. Other (optional) documents referenced as part of the process may include (3) an out-of-hospital "do not resuscitate" order, or DNR; (4), an anatomical gift donation; and (5) a durable power of attorney (with powers that go beyond the medical).

What is the purpose of each of these documents?

- **The Durable Medical Power of Attorney** permits you to appoint someone to make healthcare decisions for you if you can no longer do so yourself. These decisions include: (1) accepting or declining medical treatment; (2) terminating medical treatment; and (3) stopping or refusing to start life-sustaining treatment. This person may also be called your agent, attorney of record, attorney-in-fact, proxy, or healthcare surrogate. The document is known as a DMPA, medical power of attorney, durable power of attorney for healthcare, directive to physicians and family or surrogates, healthcare proxy, or other names.
- **A Living Will** enables you to specify your wishes regarding medical care in the event that you cannot make such decisions yourself. It may refer to receiving—or not receiving—various medical treatments under various circumstances, the intent behind those choices, and/or other details.
- **An Out-of-Hospital "Do Not Resuscitate" Order (DNR)** expresses your wish to refuse life-sustaining treatments under certain circumstances in *non-hospital* settings. These may include other types of care facilities, a hospice

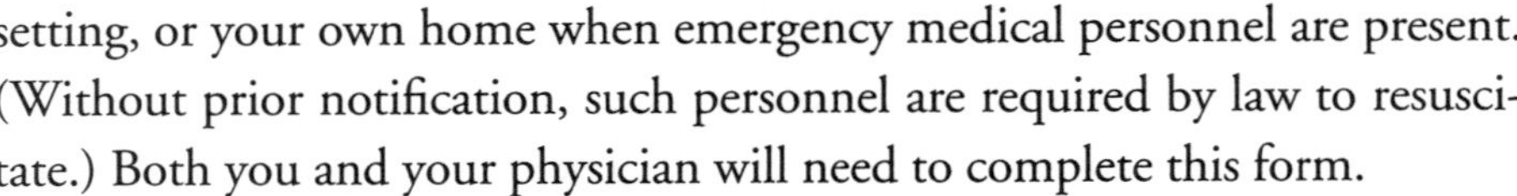

setting, or your own home when emergency medical personnel are present. (Without prior notification, such personnel are required by law to resuscitate.) Both you and your physician will need to complete this form.

- **An Anatomical Gift Donation** takes effect after your death and with it, you may (1) donate your body, organs or tissues; and/or (2) designate specific gifts for certain purposes. Valid in all fifty states, it is authorized by the Uniform Anatomical Gift Act. It does not *mandate* the donation of any part of your body after death, but it makes it an option. If you specifically do *not* want to donate, do not execute this form. Instead, discuss your wishes with your family and/or the person who holds your durable medical power of attorney.
- **A Durable Power of Attorney** grants powers beyond just the medical. It allows a designated person to carry on the financial transactions of daily living for you while you are medically incapacitated, such as signing your Social Security check, paying your bills with your checkbook, dealing with your bank, applying for disability on your behalf, and so on.

It is crucial to discuss your wishes, and the existence of these documents, with your family, friends, and loved ones—especially when you are deciding on your healthcare proxy. When choosing that person, consider that person's beliefs and definition of quality of life. Ask what that person would wish for him- or herself in a similar situation, and any other questions to help you feel confident the person will act according to your own wishes, rather than theirs.

The same goes for your choice of doctors! Ask if your doctor will honor your advance directive. If your doctor has a moral or ethical disagreement with your expressed position, the law does not compel the doctor to follow it. If your doctor, hospital, or other healthcare facility has a policy that prevents them from honoring your wishes, they must inform you in writing. If, after you are informed of their policy, you choose to continue under their care anyway, they will not be required to honor your directive.

These are not simple questions, and your views may change over time. For this reason, you need to talk to both your healthcare proxy and doctor in depth about your stated desires.

Here are a few more points to be aware of with advance directives:

- **Copies on file.** Your doctor should have a copy of your advance directive on file with your medical records. And, should life-sustaining treatment become a possibility, your doctor should forward a copy to the people and institutions involved.
- **Children.** Minor children do not need an advance directive, as their parents and legal guardians speak for them. However, if you have a terminally ill child and might have to make the excruciating decision to withhold life support, you should execute a Directive to Physicians. You may also want to execute a Standby Guardian document if, in your absence, you wish a particular person to serve as guardian.
- **Witnessing.** For documents like these, every state has some type of witnessing requirement involving one or more adults and/or a notary. Witnesses confirm that you really are the person signing the document, you are not forced to do so, and you appear to understand what you are doing. (Witnesses do not need to know the actual content of the document.) Research and follow the witnessing requirements for your state, or see an attorney.
- **Help from an attorney.** Consulting with a lawyer is always an option when considering end-of-life issues. One expert suggests it is especially advisable if (1) you live in more than one state during the course of the year; (2) you don't fully understand the standard advance directive form, or you find that it does not allow you to express your actual healthcare preferences; or (3) you have concerns that the advance directive form does not address.[1]
- **Varying state laws.** Advance directives from one state are not always valid in another. Therefore it may be safest to use the one provided by your hospital. But, since this is not always possible in an emergency, have one prepared, executed, and on file.
- **Duration and updating.** Unless specified in the document, advance directives are not null and void after any elapsed time (time-restricted directives

1 Neil J. Nusbaum, "Advance Directives," Patient Education Forum, American Geriatrics Society, http://www.americangeriatrics.org/education/forum/advance.shtml.

are a possibility). If your circumstances change—such as divorce, death of your healthcare proxy, and so on—you must change your advance directives: the newly executed one will invalidate any with a prior date. Any life change probably warrants an entirely new document, just to be safe.

Please do not let any reluctance or discomfort on your part interfere with completing and discussing these documents. They are vitally important and can save much anguish and heartache.

How do you get started? Ask your own legal advisor, or ask the hospital's legal office or patient advocacy staff: they should be able to provide you with sample documents at no charge. You will find typical examples in this book's appendix A. Use these for reference only: *do not copy* these and expect that they will comply with your state laws. You *must* seek some type of legal guidance on these documents, even if only from the hospital's legal office.

### Case Study: Access to Medical Records With and Without a DMPA

My primary legal issue during Bill's hospitalization was access to his medical information, particularly lab results.

Certainly I could make sense of lab results. With my close involvement, research, and question-asking, I became so knowledgeable that I was often asked what kind of medical training I had received. My response was usually "Twenty-four-seven since October twenty-third"—the date Bill was admitted.

But, notably, I did not have Durable Medical Power of Attorney at the beginning of Bill's hospitalization. What difference did it make? It often depended on the providers' attitudes. I have found that there are two types of providers: those who appreciate your knowledge and wish to partner with you, and those who do not. The former will often consider information access on a case-by-case basis, using common sense. The latter may adhere to "the letter of the law" every time. The real need for a DMPA occurs when you deal with the latter.

Take Hospital B, for example. For five days, the providers there denied my requests to see Bill's lab results. Whenever I sneaked a look at his labs on the table outside his room, someone removed them. So I protested, working my way up the hospital's administrative ladder until I finally reached the Patient Rights folks: the hospital office charged with advocating for patients. I now know to start there, but at that time these staff were unknown to me. It took a ninety-minute meeting, but Bill's doctor was finally convinced that I had a right to see the lab results (even though the hospital's Patient Advocacy Statement clearly specified such a right—more on that in Recommendation 5). When the doctor told me it was "unusual for a family member to want the depth of information" I sought, it seemed implausible. Hospital B was world-renowned. Most of its incoming patients and family members would be well educated about presenting conditions; they often arrived seeking alternatives.

*Take Legal Steps to Ensure the Patient's Wishes Are Honored*

Moreover, the head of the ICU required that a doctor be present while I looked at any lab results, ostensibly to explain what I did not understand. But whenever I tried to arrange such a meeting, they failed to respond. I finally asked for a set daily time for this purpose. Only on the last day of Bill's stay were his lab results shared with me in a timely fashion.

The same problem resurfaced at Hospital C, to a lesser extent. But when I was denied lab result access upon entry at Hospital D, I decided the time had come. Bill was now mentally competent, so I asked his attorney friend Skip to draft both a Durable Medical Power of Attorney and a living will.

When I presented them to Bill, I told him I thought we were past needing these, but let's not take any chances. Bill made minor revisions, we found witnesses, and we both cried as we executed the documents. An attorney from the hospital's legal department accepted service—officially acknowledged their receipt. I made multiple copies and kept both documents in my purse.

Less than three weeks later, Bill coded—seizures and a stroke—and returned to the medical ICU, unconscious and on full life support. We were uncertain what his mental condition would be upon waking. so the living will could easily have been essential. Thankfully, we did not need it.

But I used my copy of the Durable Medical Power of Attorney many times. From that time on, whenever I had a problem with information access, I produced it and that resolved the issue. How I wish we had executed one before Bill was admitted to Hospital A.

## *Checklist E: Preparing Legal Documents*

*Take Legal Steps to Ensure the Patient's Wishes Are Honored*

| STEPS TO TAKE | ✓ |
|---|---|
| **For Durable Medical Power of Attorney and/or a living will (sometimes merged as one document, often called an advance directive)** | |
| Obtain a sample Durable Medical Power of Attorney document and a sample living will. | |
| Make revisions to the Durable Medical Power of Attorney and living will only with appropriate counsel. | |
| Type and print at least four originals of each. | |
| Execute all originals in blue ink (to distinguish originals from copies), complying with requirements for witness[es] and notary signatures. | |
| Make at least four photocopies of each. | |
| Serve the hospital legal office or administration with one **original** of the Durable Medical Power of Attorney document and one **original** of the living will. Receive proof-of-service acknowledgements for each document from hospital and place in safekeeping. | |
| Retain an **original of each** to be carried on your person, place one **copy** of each in the hands of the hospital's Patient Rights advocate, and place the remaining **originals** in safekeeping (such as a safety deposit box or fireproof vault). Keep remaining copies at home, easily accessible. | |
| **For Power of Attorney (going beyond the medical)** | |
| Obtain a sample Power of Attorney document. | |
| Make revisions to the Power of Attorney only with appropriate counsel. | |
| Type and print at least four originals. | |
| Execute all originals in blue ink (to distinguish originals from copies), complying with requirements for witness[es] and notary signatures. | |
| Make at least four copies. | |
| Serve any bank or business with an **original** Power of Attorney to enable you to take legal actions. Receive proof-of-service acknowledgement from the receiving party and place in safekeeping. | |
| Retain an **original** to be carried on your person and place remaining **originals** in safekeeping (such as a safety deposit box or fireproof vault). Keep remaining copies at home, easily accessible. | |

recommendation
5

# READ AND USE THE *Patient Advocacy Statement*

THIS IS PARTICULARLY true when you have been granted Durable Medical Power of Attorney. Ask what the rules are and challenge any that don't make sense to you.

*With a stout heart, a mouse can lift an elephant.*
—TIBETAN PROVERB

*Read and Use the Patient Advocacy Statement*

We live in the information age. In our era, in our time and place, knowledge is the true currency of personal power—more than muscle, more than land ownership, even more than monetary wealth. If you want more power, you will need more knowledge.

Remember this as a patient advocate. Here, too, information is power. One of our best tools is this: know your patient's rights and hold hospitals accountable to them. Hospitals do acknowledge that patients have specific rights—at least in theory. So make sure both you and your loved one know about them.

## The Patient Advocacy Statement: What Is It?

Usually, upon admission, all patients receive a copy of the hospital's own Patient Advocacy Statement, often called a Patient Rights Statement. The content of this "bill of rights" varies from hospital to hospital. But it generally states that patients can expect certain practices and standards during their stay: rights pertaining to issues such as privacy, safety, decision making, access to information, and quality of care. It may also state the patient's responsibilities, such as providing complete information, following rules and treatment plans, and so on. It may provide other information, too: for example, it may explain the role of the staff patient advocate and the hospital's grievance protocols. Make sure both you and your loved one have a copy of your hospital's Patient Advocacy Statement, and read it in full. For a preview of a typical statement, see this book's appendix B.

Whenever you read such a statement, do so with a critical eye. Although they are framed as rights and responsibilities, these rules exist primarily for the hospital's own protection. As Bill pointed out to me later, "Rules are generally made in response to litigation." Whether as a result of lawsuits or not, hospitals have found it advantageous to frame these expectations explicitly. Yes, these rules can serve the patient, but they also serve the hospital. It's up to you to make sure they serve your loved one.

### *Rights that deal with decision making and information access*

The seven patient rights listed below are key ones for advocates, I have found, because they deal with decision making and information access. These are drawn from the example in appendix B. But remember: your hospital's statement will likely differ from this one, so read it in full.



The patient has the right to:

- Appoint a surrogate to make healthcare decisions on your behalf to the extent permitted by law.
- Understandable information concerning diagnosis, treatment and prognosis, and financial implications of treatment choices.
- Involvement in medical decision-making, including refusal of care and treatment, to the extent permitted by law, and being informed of the medical consequences of refusal.
- Reasonable access to review medical records pertaining to your care, and to receive copies of these records for a reasonable photocopying fee.
- Be informed of and participate in treatment decisions and the care planning process.
- Be informed of hospital policies and resources, such as Patient Rights advocates and the ethics committee.
- Expect a reasonable response to your need/request for assistance in effective communication, regardless of language or disability.

These sound positive—but be wary. Just because the rules exist doesn't mean hospitals always comply. They don't. And if they don't, call them on it. The tips below, gleaned from my own experience, all illustrate hospital noncompliance in the information sphere.

A few tips for protecting your information rights:

- *Ask about the library and other information resources.* Not one of the four hospitals told me about the in-hospital library available to me.

*Read and Use the Patient Advocacy Statement*

- *Be aware of distraction techniques; they may indicate withheld information.* In Hospital B, after I objected twice to Bill's treatment with a strong psychotropic drug, the chair of the psych department came to talk to me. But rather than address my concerns about the drug, she diverted the conversation: How was I? Was I taking care of myself? Good questions, under other circumstances, but here she was simply trying to derail my complaint.
- *Insist on access to the information you need.* I was often denied access to Bill's hospital records: information I needed in order to act on his behalf.
- *Ask for information about the patient advocate on staff.* Not one of the four hospitals told me about this resource, or about a patient's right to challenge hospital employees' actions. (As a result, I almost lost unrestricted access to Bill at Hospital D—more on that story later.)

When the patient is out of commission, as Bill was, advocates may struggle to get access to medical records and treatment plans—especially if they have not been granted Durable Medical Power of Attorney. In that case, hospitals must balance the patient's right to confidentiality against the advocate's right to the information needed to act on a patient's behalf. Federal laws on patient privacy may further complicate the issue. But as advocates, we often find ourselves pressing for information. That is part of our role. Here are five points to remember:

1. We must be willing to engage in conflict.
2. We must do our homework so we know what quesions to ask.
3. We must be assertive, even with busy doctors and nurses.
4. We must be willing to ask specialists about side effects and other effects of their treatments.
5. We must make extra effort to talk with doctors who—as many do—have trouble communicating, even if they are gifted technicians.

As an advocate for your loved one, you either have to speak up or get help with these issues. Check your own Patient Advocacy Statement for the relevant items, and refer to them as needed.

### *Other patient rights: A few examples*

The rights listed in your Patient Advocacy Statement may range widely, from the specific to the general. Here are a few examples, together with my comments on our personal experience.

The patient has a right to:

- *Be free from restraints or seclusion, imposed as a means of coercion, discipline, convenience or retaliation by staff.* I found that all four hospitals were careful with this one. At one point Bill did need to be restrained—he was confused and often pulled out tubes—and the nurses were very diligent about discussing this with me in advance.
- *Confidentiality of information.* Sometimes I felt the care providers were trying to keep information about Bill's condition so confidential that it was off limits even from me! One hospital employee even said as much to me.
- *Decline participation in experimental treatments.* In Hospital D, Bill had the option of joining an experimental protocol for treating bedsores. I was asked if I wanted Bill to participate or simply try the new treatment. I chose the latter.

Be aware, too, that patient rights may differ on the psychiatric unit. Hospitals often use the term "lock-up" to describe their method of ensuring patient safety here. If your loved one will be in this unit, even if only briefly, ask how the rules differ from other areas of the hospital.

## Don't Count on Staff Patient Advocates: A Cautionary Tale

Hospitals may tout their own staff advocates as protectors of your rights, but remember that these people are hospital employees. During Bill's stay at Hospital D, a staff advocate got involved in a problem that arose—but I found that person to be of no help. In fact, she sided with the hospital. The problem actually threatened my participation in Bill's care, so it is worth repeating here as a cautionary tale.

5

*Read and Use the Patient Advocacy Statement*

By the time Bill was in the Hospital D's medical intensive care unit (MICU), I knew a lot about his care and the equipment involved, including the ventilator that kept him breathing. In fact, the nurses and therapists had often asked me to assist in his room. Staff had shown me, for example, how to temporarily silence the ventilator alarm. I had done this frequently when staff couldn't respond right away: I shut it off, then pressed the call button and looked for a nurse to come to the bedside.

One day as I was turning off the alarm after three minutes of chiming, the respiratory therapist entered and told me I was not to touch the equipment. She said that she herself was responsible for managing the ventilator and its alarm: that was true. When I told her about the many times I had done this in the past, and why, she said she didn't care—I was not to touch the ventilator. She then reported me to the head nurse, I learned later.

The next day, with Bill's mother also in the room, I was helping a nurse change Bill's bedding when the alarm rang again, as it often does when the patient is rolled. The nurse asked me to silence it and, since I was on that side of the bed, I reached over and shut it off. Just then, a staff member in the hall glanced into the room. From that angle, only I and the ventilator were visible, but not the nurse. Apparently my actions were immediately reported to the head nurse who, upon arriving at work the next day, asked me to leave Bill's room. My mother-and-law and I waited in an adjacent "quiet room" for about an hour. Then the head nurse returned with this verdict: because I was "intentionally interfering with my husband's treatment"—touching the ventilator—I was now denied access to his room. I would be allowed only when a staff member was present.

Outraged and upset, I wasn't sure where to turn. Luckily, a visitor had just arrived: Lee, one of Bill's respiratory therapists from Hospital A. She was appalled at my story and called a nurse colleague, Rebecca, who also knew us well. Rebecca came to my rescue, going straight to the hospital's Patient Advocacy Office and asking for an immediate hearing. So, while I was still crying in the MICU hallway, several employees—the head nurse, a Patient Rights advocate, a social worker, and a hospital attorney—met to prepare for my hearing. When they finally invited me to join them, I brought my mother-in-law, Lee, and Rebecca for support.

The head nurse leveled his charge—"intentionally interfering" with the treatment—then proceeded to talk nonstop until even his colleagues asked him to let me tell my side of the story. I did, and I also asked whether the head nurse had talked to the nurse who asked me to silence the alarm (he had not). My supporters then verified that I knew what I was doing. Never had I interfered with Bill's treatment.

5

*Read and Use the Patient Advocacy Statement*

Although I could see that our words were having an impact, I could also see that the hospital wasn't about to lift the ban. Here, I would have expected some mediation from the staff advocate—but she was silent. So I played my trump card, as Rebecca had suggested: if I was denied access to Bill, I would seriously consider filing a malpractice suit against the hospital.

Boy, did that get their attention! Suddenly, the heretofore silent attorney sat up straighter, asked me what I meant, and started taking copious notes. So I made my case—my presence was an asset. In fact, I had twice averted distaster: I noticed a loose tube after Bill had been dropped during a transfer, and I was there when a mis-set monitor failed to notify the nurse that his heart was racing: sinus ventricular tachychardia.

It was amazing how soon after that I was granted unrestricted access to Bill. Later I learned that the head nurse was demoted for his role in this travesty.

The incident was resolved, but let's note several things about it. First, the hospital staff stuck together, including the so-called patient advocate. Second, I learned about the appeal process only through Rebecca: no staff had told me about it. And third—incidental to the problem, but worth noting—I knew about Bill's transfer drop and the mis-set monitor only because I was present 24/7.

All the participants visited me later and apologized for how things were handled. Was this true remorse or lawsuit prevention? I will never know. But among other things, I had learned to be wary of staff patient advocates.

## Federal Laws on Confidentiality: What They Mean to You

In 2003, Congress passed new legislation to tighten up confidentiality in healthcare as part of the Health Insurance Portability and Accountability Act of 1996, affectionately called HIPAA. According to a press release, this legislation was designed to "reassure patients of the confidentiality of their medical records . . . [and give them] greater access and more control over . . . [the] personal information . . . in their own medical records."[1] Healthcare industry leaders did not try to block this legislation because they thought its passage would ease the introduction of computerized patient records (a tool that fewer than 25 percent of U.S. doctors had implemented as of September 2006).[2]



During Bill's hospitalization in 2000 and 2001, before the HIPAA legislation, I had to fight to get information about his condition. If I had this kind of difficulty without the presence of these supposed protections, what might I expect today? Subsequent to his discharge, I have discovered that healthcare facilities tend to err on the side of "too much" patient privacy rather than "not enough." While violators do not appear to be treated harshly, as with other laws, many hospitals have gone to the extreme in enforcement, so much so that the legal profession has crafted a document designed to "override" the protections put in place. To get certain types of information, family members must release the hospital from damages by signing a legal doscument called the HIPAA Medical Information Release Form. (See its text in appendix A.) And remember, both the patient and the advocate are in serious trouble these days if no Durable Medical Power of Attorney has been granted.

Let's review the HIPAA statement of one of the hospitals where Bill stayed.

### *The Medical Information and Privacy Statement*

This statement is one hospital's response to the 2003 HIPAA leigslation and governs how, and to whom, hospitals release information. The Medical Information and Privacy Statement—often many pages long—also varies from hospital to hospital. Yours will probably look similar to the sample in appendix B.

During Bill's illness the Medical Information and Privacy Statement was not part of hospital protocol, so I cannot vouch for its usefulness. But, like the Patient Advocacy Statement, it bears scrutiny.

---

1 Phoenix Health Systems, "HHS Secretary Thompson and the Press: On Reaching the Privacy Deadline," HIPAAdvisory.com, April 14, 2003 http://www.hipaadvisory.com/alert/vol4/news041403.htm.

2 Steven Reinberg, "U.S. Health-Care System Scores a D for Quality."

In the three excerpts below, the issue is control over disclosure of medical records. (Note especially the bolded words: this language makes it even more imperative that your loved one execute a Durable Medical Power of Attorney.)

- *We* ***may*** *disclose medical information about you to a friend or family member who is involved in your care.*
- *Unless you object, we* ***may*** *disclose medical information about you to a friend or family member who is involved in your medical care and we may disclose medical information about you to an entity assisting in a disaster relief effort so that your family can be notified about your location and condition.*
- ***If you are not present or able to object, then we may, using our professional judgment, determine whether the disclosure is in your best interest.***

Read and Use the Patient Advocacy Statement

Another area of concern: family access to the medical information used to make decisions. Although the statement below says the *patient* has the right to see such records, it is silent regarding family members or advocates.

- *Right to Inspect and Copy. You have the right to inspect and have copied medical information used to make decisions about your care. Usually, this includes medical and billing records, but does not include some records such as psychotherapy notes.*

And the following statement is silent on timeliness:

- *To inspect and have copied medical information used to make decisions about you, you must submit your request in writing. Call Release of Information at [number] for further details. We may charge a fee for the costs of processing your request.*

For me, the lack of time frame made this "right" moot. Because Hospital B had made it so hard for me to see Bill's X rays and CT scans, I asked the staff to forward copies to me when we left so I could share them with his next healthcare team. The requested films did not show up until a year later—obviously, too late to be useful.

Now let's look at the other side of the coin: do you want to specifically *exclude* anyone from receiving information? The next excerpt speaks to that.

*Read and Use the Patient Advocacy Statement*

- *Right to Request Restrictions. You have the right to request a restriction or limitation on the medical information we use or disclose about you for treatment, payment or healthcare operations. You also have the right to request a limit on the medical information we disclose about you to someone who is involved in your care or in the payment for your care, like a family member or friend.* ***We are not required to agree to your request.*** *If we do agree, we will comply with your request unless the information is needed to provide you emergency treatment.*

Again, my personal experience illustrates the issue. In Bill's case, one particular former family member made herself unwelcome. She called Hospital A frequently while Bill was comatose, often occupying his nurse on the phone for twenty minutes at a time. Despite our pleas to ask Bill's family for updates, rather than distracting Bill's nurses, she continued to call. At that point, I asked that the hospital refuse to give her information, since she had no legal right to it. Next, she "pretended to be someone else on the phone," one nurse told us. And when she finally threatened to sue for withholding relevant information, the hospital gave her the information.

This scenario was repeated at the next two hospitals, and they, too, capitulated to her (groundless) lawsuit threat and supplied whatever data she requested—despite her non-family status. Only Hospital D told her that no details would be forthcoming and she could file suit if she chose.

Would a Medical Information and Privacy Statement have helped us here? Could we then have insisted that the first three hospitals not release information to her? Maybe, but I can't be sure—partly because the law only allows the *patient* to stop the information flow; it doesn't specifically grant that right to a patient advocate. Moreover, note the bolded passage in the above excerpt: the hospital reserves the right to make its own judgment call regarding this issue.

The bottom line is this: patient treatment information is getting harder to access without legal authority. Access rules are now federally regulated, to some extent, so you must play by the rules. If you haven't been granted Durable Medical Power of Attorney, but you need access to certain protected records, the hospital's Patient Rights Office may be able to help. Do seek help there, but keep possible conflicts of interest in mind. You can also seek legal counsel yourself.

And, if you must fight, remember Helen Keller's words: "I am only one; but still I am one. I cannot do everything, but still I can do something; I will not refuse to do something I can do."

*Read and Use the Patient Advocacy Statement*

As groundwork for your patient's rights, first help the providers see your loved one as a real person. Bring in photos of the person in good health and post them in the room. To the providers at the bedside, the person suddenly becomes more real: real because the healthy appearance offers a goal; real because we see family and friends who care deeply; real because the person clearly has a life to which he or she wants to return. I posted pictures on Bill's door to show his providers what he looked like vertical! Although that became a good-natured joke, those pictures served a serious purpose. They represented a defining moment—an unconscious patient became a real human being to his healthcare team. Then, and only then, could I begin to deal with Bill's and my rights.

*recommendation*
6

# ASSUME YOUR LOVED ONE CAN HEAR EVERYTHING, *so Speak in the Positive*

We are told that people in a coma can hear what we say, even if they cannot respond. So make your words affirmative. This is also a good idea when you are talking to the universe—or to God.

*A strong positive attitude will create more miracles than any wonder drug.*
—Patricia Neal

*Assume Your Loved One Can Hear Everything, so Speak in the Positive*

In his book *Awaken to the Healer Within*, Rich Work discusses what he calls the universal laws that govern all creation. Here are the first two (a third will be discussed in Recommendation 13):

> ***The Law of Magnetic Attraction***
> *You attract to you that which you desire. You also attract to you that which you do not desire—if you focus on it. If you focus on disease, you will manifest more disease. If you focus on poverty, you will manifest more poverty. If you focus on the lack of love in your life, you will only manifest more lack. It is not possible to create love when you focus on fear. It is not possible to create prosperity when you focus on poverty. That is the Law of Magnetic Attraction.*
>
> ***The Law of Creative Manifestation***
> *Now that you understand law 1, invoke law 2. Intentionally focus on that which you desire. And, do not focus on that which you do not desire in your life. If you are in a room where others are engaged in a conversation about something that you do not desire, politely excuse yourself and leave. To remain in that energy will only attract more of it into your life.*[1]

My interpretation of these laws, coupled with my own experience, revealed this to me: Bill heard everything during his illness, even while he was in a coma. During that time I noticed that sensitive doctors stepped outside Bill's room to discuss his (grim) condition. The insensitive ones began talking right there at Bill's side. If the gist was negative and I was present, I asked to move the conversation outside the room. Those who saw me as a partner complied. Those who didn't usually gave a reply such as "Your husband has a right to hear about his condition." While I agree with that in theory, circumstances also play a role. If a patient is anesthetized, unconscious, and critically ill, it is not helpful to tell him that his chance of surviving surgery is less than 5 percent. Avoid whispered conversations in a patient's presence, too. The whispers suggest something withheld.

Early in his recovery at home, Bill took a two-week trip to his mother's home in Florida. During the visit, he and his mom discussed his hospitalization in

1 Rich Work with Ann Marie Groth, *Awaken to the Healer Within*, 23–24.

detail, and as a result of some of their conversations, he came home concluding that "I think I heard my mom when I was unconscious in the hospital."

This conclusion came nine months after his discharge from the hospital. Whether it was actually true or he simply wished it so, the fact is that Bill's mother and I constantly spoke positively to him while he was hospitalized. Every day, I wrote and posted an affirmation on the wall for him to see: "My kidneys are healthy," for example, or "I can and will walk up and down the hall today."

Bill's primary in-hospital physical therapist, Lori, also wrote affirmations and posted progress charts for him to see. During his crucial septic episodes, all of us involved took turns holding Bill's hand and telling him how much we wanted him to stay. Even though he was unconscious at the time, perhaps he chose to stay because he heard us. In any case, he survived against all odds.

Every time a negative statement was made or negative event happened in his room or within his hearing, Bill had some kind of setback. Twice I had heated discussions with doctors in his room—I was tired and didn't think to move into the hall. Both times Bill had physical or mental setbacks afterward.

My friend Jean, a Reiki master who did energy work with Bill daily for two months, taught me that the universe may hear our words differently than we speak them. If we say "I don't want to feel pain today," the universe translates this into "I feel pain today." Negatives don't register, so why use them? State everything in the positive, as if it were so. The universe will respond to align the words and the wish—as when Captain Picard of the starship *Enterprise* said, "Make it so!" and Wesley Crusher promptly complied.

Said another way, using affirmations is like taking the psychologist's advice: "'Act as if' and it will become so." Think of specific affirmations for your situation and write them down, but also look at the many books and card decks that contain affirmations. Use your local bookstore or library. You can also find Internet sites that offer health-related affirmations, some of which may be very specific to the condition of your loved one.

Change starts inside. Positive words begin to affect our thoughts, our thoughts affect our behavior, and eventually it all affects our "outer packaging"—our body. Try these affirmations:

- I have the power to control my health.
- I am in control of my health and wellness.
- I have abundant energy, vitality, and well-being.
- I am healthy in all aspects of my being.



If you create a positive environment for healing, healing is much more likely to take place. As Mahatma Gandhi said, "Be the change you want to see in the world."

recommendation
7

# EDUCATE *Yourself*

Learn all you can about your loved one's illness or injury and its treatment. The more you know, the more you can help the healthcare providers—even if you have to win them over first. Medical technology is invaluable, but some providers rely so heavily on it that they fail to look at the patient.

*The real voyage of discovery consists not in seeking new landscapes, but in having new eyes.*
—Marcel Proust

Once we've begun to state everything in the positive, we can start learning more about the specifics of the challenge facing us and our loved one. Be as fully informed as you can. Attitude is important, but so are knowledge and understanding. A story passed around the Internet illustrates this point:

7

*Educate Yourself*

> Many years ago, when I worked as a volunteer at a hospital, I got to know a little girl named Liz, who was suffering from a rare and serious disease. Her only chance of recovery appeared to be a blood transfusion from her five-year-old brother, who had miraculously survived the same disease and had developed the antibodies needed to combat the illness.
>
> The doctor explained the situation to her little brother, and asked the little boy if he would be willing to give his blood to his sister. I saw him hesitate for only a moment before taking a deep breath and saying, "Yes, I'll do it if it will save her."
>
> As the transfusion progressed, he lay in bed next to his sister and smiled, as we all did, seeing the color returning to her cheeks. Then his face grew pale and his smile faded. He looked up at the doctor and asked with a trembling voice, "Will I start to die right away?"
>
> Being young, the little boy had misunderstood the doctor; he thought he was going to have to give his sister all of his blood in order to save her. You see, after all, understanding and attitude are everything.[1]

So let's learn! Start with the obvious: learn the names of your care providers, and treat them with respect and appreciation. Bill's nurses were always grateful for the small favors I'd bring them, such as cookies, candy, and doughnuts. Establish appreciative relationships with care providers and they will naturally be more willing to help you.

Ask them questions about everything. A respectful tone will get you a more complete response. For example, "Can you help me understand . . . ?" served me well as an opener. I kept a notebook with me and wrote down the information I received and who said it. Then, when I had questions for another doctor about the same subject, I could quote both the statement and the source from a prior discussion. Be advised: there will be days when the doctors won't have time to

---

1 Anonymous, "Five Important Lessons," Inspire21.com, http://www.inspire21.com/site/stories/05-Stories/five_lessons.html.

talk with you or won't wish to do so. In such cases, see if they can tell you when they will have time or whether another source, such as a medical resident or student, can serve the same purpose. Don't take no for an answer. Not only do you have a right to know what is going on and to understand the treatment to the best of your ability, you are paying for the service! The doctors and nurses work for you and your loved one. They are not doing you a favor! Remember the Patient Advocacy Statement: you are entitled to "understandable information concerning diagnosis, treatment and prognosis, and financial implications of treatment choices."

Another source of information is the hospital library. All hospitals have one, although you may have to ask where to find it. As with any library, some books may be removed and others may not. A photocopier should be available for copying the relevant material from books that cannot be removed; most libraries allow up to a certain number of free copies. If you lack computer access to search the Internet at the hospital, some medical libraries may grant you online access and even help you with your search. This is more likely in a teaching or university hospital library, less likely in a private one. Regardless, it doesn't hurt to ask.

The Internet is a rich source of information. But choose reliable websites: because the Internet is not regulated, some sites may have information that is outdated, inaccurate, and potentially harmful. Check some of the sites in the Resources section of this book for starters. When I was researching Bill's medical conditions, the Web was my best source for up-to-date information and treatment protocols. Some of the material was so good that Bill's doctors asked for copies of the articles!

An underused but valuable resource is the literature found on the hospital units themselves. In Hospital A, I found an exhaustive nurse's text that supplied a great deal of information on care and disease. On every floor of every hospital we were in, I found a *Physicians' Desk Reference*. Among other things, the *PDR* has detailed information on drugs, their purposes, and their side effects. I relied on it heavily when new medications were prescribed for Bill. Did I understand all the technical language? No, but I gleaned enough knowledge that I could intelligently voice my concerns, or my support, to the doctors during their rounds.

*The Pill Book*, or any similar drug reference guide that is published yearly, will serve the same purpose.

I always looked at the contraindications of specific drugs—that is, conditions under which they should not be given—and their potential interactions with other drugs. Because I was concerned was the impact of Bill's medications on his kidneys—a vulnerable spot for him—I also carefully noted what organs were involved in the breakdown and absorption of each medicine. Several times I brought up the topic of the kidneys' role in processing a certain drug and asked doctors to consider alternatives. Know your loved one's key vulnerabilities, and focus your efforts there at first. You can then expand your field of focus.

Despite my eagerness to learn, I was often frightened by my research. When an article described the progression of acute pancreatitis and offered survival rates based on certain factors, I assessed the factors against Bill's condition. More often than not, they pointed to death. Although this scared me, at least I understood the extent of his illness. And I increased the frequency and intensity of my prayers.

With regard to your loved one's illness, disease, or injury, ignorance is not bliss. Advocacy is a labor of love, and anything you can face, you can handle. Arming yourself with knowledge shows that you expect to be taken seriously. Part of your role is to pay attention to the whole patient: this is especially critical in the "body part specialty" hospitals—teaching or university hospitals—where you may be the only one who takes that role.

Learn about the equipment and technology used in treatment, too. According to Confucius, "The beginning of wisdom is to call things by their right names." At the very least, know the name and purpose of each machine and monitor at the bedside. Many are set to ring an alarm under certain conditions. If an alarm rings and you need to notify a nurse, using the right terms will get your message across quickly and clearly.

Even if you have no medical background, plunge right in. Now is the time to begin your education! You will gain credibility with physicians and other staff if you can speak their language, even just a little. Doors will open—with doctors, with nurses, and with your loved one, who will want to understand and may rely on you to translate.

*recommendation*
8

# ASK ABOUT EVERY *Medication, Injection, and IV Solution*

GUARD YOUR PATIENT'S safety by helping monitor the administration of drugs and other fluids—and keep side effects in mind.

*When we try to pick out anything by itself, we find it hitched to everything else in the universe.*
—JOHN MUIR

# 8

## *Ask About Every Medication, Injection, and IV Solution*

There are five rules for the correct administration of drugs:

- right patient
- right drug
- right dose
- right route
- right time[1]

That goes for injections, medicines in any form, drug and non-drug solutions given through intravenous (IV) lines—any deliberate introduction of a treatment-related substance into the patient's body.

Hospital patients wear wristbands showing their name and listing any allergies. Staff members who administer drugs should always check the wristband first. This does not always happen, and it can lead to mistakes.

As patient advocates, we can help. We can post a sign by the bed listing our loved one's name, room number, bed number (if the room is shared), allergies, chronic conditions, and impairments (such as sight or hearing). That's one simple thing we can do to improve the odds in our patient's favor—and it's especially important if the person is unconscious.

As a nation, the United States has a high instance of medical errors (including medication errors) compared with some of its industrialized counterparts. In a 2005 study that also included Australia, Canada, Germany, New Zealand, and the United Kingdom, 34 percent of the U.S. healthcare workers surveyed reported such errors, the highest rate of all six nations. The survey is conducted annually by the Commonwealth Fund International Health Policy Survey.[2] Let's try to bring that percentage down.

---

1 California Department of Developmental Services, "Nursing Medication Training Program Plan," CA.gov, http://www.dds.ca.gov/ICF/PDF/ICF_DDN/DDN_MedTrainingPlan.pdf.

2 Commonwealth Fund, "Health System Views and Experiences Among Sicker Adults in Six Countries."

Keeping these five rules in mind, let's look at how we can advocate for our patient most effectively, starting with medications in general, and then considering the particular pros and cons of IV lines.

## Medications

*Ask About Every Medication, Injection, and IV Solution*

Keep a close eye on what your loved one is prescribed and whether is is administered as directed. And, if it is denied or discontinued, find out why. There may be more to it than meets the eye. You may know a key detail that the healthcare provider does not know. This story illustrates several mishaps that an advocate can help solve.

It was 1:15 AM during our seventh month in the hospital. On a cot at my husband's side, I woke up wondering if he had received one of his medications that night, an antidepressant. Because the delivery system for this drug was experimental—a gel that crosses the skin-blood barrier—I was quite sure he had not: I would have seen the nurse apply it to his arm.

I approached the nurse and asked if Bill had received the antidepressant that evening. She looked blank and told me she didn't remember seeing it on the MARS—the Medication Administration Record Sheet. So I asked her to check. What a surprise! It was on the MARS, but she had overlooked it. She had signed off indicating that she had given it to Bill, because it was supposed to have been included in a batch of drugs she picked up at the pharmacy earlier. But it wasn't. No internal alarm went off because she had never given this drug by the gel route before. She apologized profusely and called the pharmacy.

Five minutes later, she was back in Bill's room telling me there was a problem. No gel compound had been prepared, and the pharmacist on duty did not know how to mix it. Bill would have to wait until the next day, when someone else could mix it for him.

The words I used in response to this explanation are unprintable. Suffice it to say I found it unacceptable. I asked the nurse to call the pharmacist back and ask three questions:

- Since when can the pharmacy service override the orders of an attending physician?

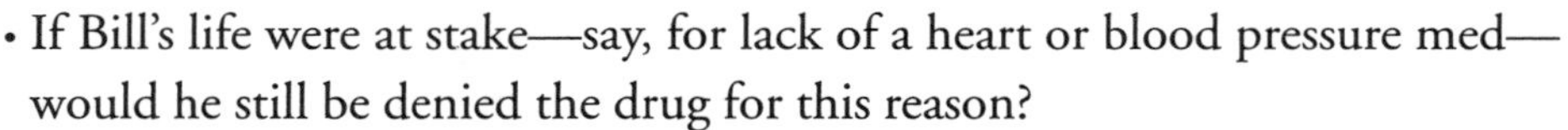
- If Bill's life were at stake—say, for lack of a heart or blood pressure med—would he still be denied the drug for this reason?

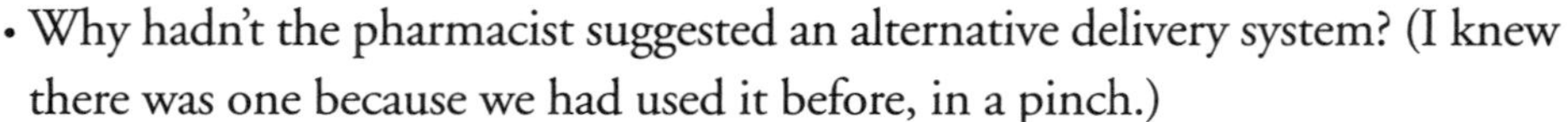
- Why hadn't the pharmacist suggested an alternative delivery system? (I knew there was one because we had used it before, in a pinch.)

*Ask About Every Medication, Injection, and IV Solution*

Another surprise! Ten minutes later the pharmacist called back: he had found some gel. The nurse could pick up the medication for immediate use. I took a tranquilizer and went to sleep. Another crisis averted, but too close for comfort. Had I not challenged the omission, Bill would have failed to receive his medication that night.

The next morning during his rounds with his staff, Bill's primary doctor asked me, "How did last night go?" and I shared this story. At that point a medical resident told me that because the drug in question stays in the system for twenty-four hours, Bill would have been OK even without it.

What's wrong with this answer?

Had she reviewed Bill's chart before her rounds, she would have known that for Bill, the stakes were high if this antidepressant were thrown off schedule. Bill had been taking it for six years, but it had been temporarily discontinued during his last episode in the ICU. (This was legitimate, as it can react adversely with other drugs, although I wished I'd been told at the time.) Now we were in the process of "titrating"—that is, tapering back up to a therapeutic dosage. That process should not be interrupted, especially for a long-term user: the drug's benefits can be seriously compromised.

How did I know these facts? Earlier, when the medication was stopped under similar circumstances in Hospital B, Bill's symptoms had begun to reappear, and I had talked to the pharmacist there. In all, this drug was stopped and restarted a total of four times during his illness. Guess who was responsible for pointing out the problem with the stoppage and asking the doctors to restart it? His advocate—me.

A dear friend's mother, also with pancreatitis, had a similar story. Like Bill, she was also labeled NPO (nothing by mouth) upon admittance, so several of her oral medications were stopped. Three of these were for psychiatric management, and she had been on them for more than twenty years. Each was labeled with a warning: "If you suddenly stop taking this drug, you may experience withdrawal symptoms." The fourth was a beta-blocker to regulate her heart rate. Guess what happened after her admission? Within twenty-four hours she had withdrawal symptoms; within forty-eight her heart was in hyperdrive, beating over 170 times a minute. As her patient advocate, I had my hands full.



Bring your knowledge of the patient's history to every conversation with healthcare providers, and don't hesitate to point out potential problems.

Even with no extenuating circumstances, medicines can simply get overlooked. It was a recurrent problem with the medication for Bill's bedsores, which were excruciatingly painful. Nurses were to apply a topical morphine regularly to ease the pain. And yet it was often overlooked.

Hold hospitals to their word about pain management. Lately hospitals have become more proactive in this area, asking both adult and child patients to rate their pain level on a scale such as the FACES scale shown here (used with permission). Staff in all four of Bill's hospitals were specially trained on this topic, and posters appeared proclaiming the patient's right to pain medication and describing pain assessment. Is there a disparity between your hospital's words and its actions? If so, step in.

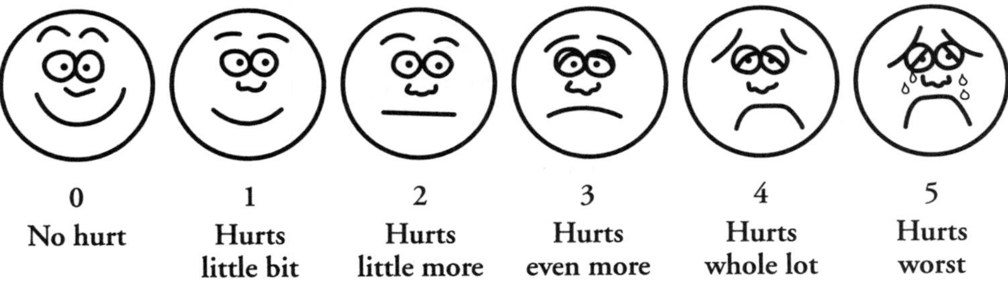

| 0 | 1 | 2 | 3 | 4 | 5 |
|---|---|---|---|---|---|
| **No hurt** | **Hurts little bit** | **Hurts little more** | **Hurts even more** | **Hurts whole lot** | **Hurts worst** |

In brief: when your patient is about to be given a medication, always ask what it is and what it is for. Notice any changes in the regimen and inquire if you don't understand it fully. Notice not only what is prescribed, but what is discontinued, withheld, or denied. Don't hesitate to ask or object. There is little emotional consolation in a malpractice lawsuit.

## A Higher-Risk Route: Intravenous Lines and Other Ports

*Ask About Every Medication, Injection, and IV Solution*

Intravenous lines are a standard, common part of modern medicine. Recall the five rules at the beginning of this chapter: IV lines are a "route" into the body. Through these narrow tubes, or lines, a liquid solution gradually enters the body through a tiny opening in a vein, often in the arm, usually made with a needle. Sometimes a special device or "port" is placed at the opening. The "IV pole" often seen at the hospital bedside usually has a bag of intravenous solution hanging from it: this liquid is steadily "dripped" into the bloodstream, and it should be painless for the patient. IV solutions don't only serve to administer drugs: they may carry nutrution to the bloodstream, help hydrate the body with a saline solution, or serve numerous other purposes. Giving IV solutions to dehydrated or undernourished patients is considered a routine practice in hospitals. It may be routine but that doesn't make it safe!

Keep this in mind: IV lines are often a necessity, but every time the hospital "punches a hole" in your loved one, the possibility of infection increases. According to a 2006 Mayo Clinic news release, "all types of catheters and other devices that allow access to the bloodstream . . . [also called] 'intravascular devices' (IVDs) have become the leading cause of bloodstream infections in the United States and worldwide . . . In the United States, as many as 500,000 IVD-related bloodstream infections occur each year, resulting in increased patient health problems and prolonged hospital stays."[3]

As noted above, other types of entry into the body also carry these risks. Catheters, drainage tubes, feeding tubes into the stomach, dialysis ports: all serve crucial purposes, but all should be carefully maintained and monitored.

The problem is, these avenues tend to invite the stuff on the outside of the body to get inside where it doesn't belong. We all have invisible intruders living on our skin: germs, bacteria, and so on. Outside the body or in the nose, they do little harm. But when you open a pathway for some other purpose, and these intruders find their way in, they have the potential to do dastardly damage to our innards. They might enter during the actual "needlestick" or original

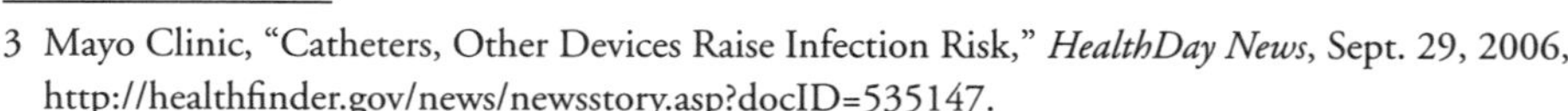

3 Mayo Clinic, "Catheters, Other Devices Raise Infection Risk," *HealthDay News*, Sept. 29, 2006, http://healthfinder.gov/news/newsstory.asp?docID=535147.

incision; they might find their way in if the line, tube, catheter, or other device isn't kept clean or gets contaminated.

When an IV line gets infected, the bad guys enter the bloodstream and travel to all parts of the body. This kind of pervasive blood infection is called sepsis, characterized by raging fever, low blood pressure, and increased respiration. (Toxic shock syndrome, caused by wearing tampons for too long, is a recognized form of sepsis.) Sepsis is life-threatening! And of Bill's thirteen septic episodes in the hospital, all but one were caused by IV line infections. Two were especially bad, with his blood pressure hovering arount 60/30 for several hours, and simultaneous heart attacks and strokes. Granted, he was critically ill and highly susceptible to such infections; moreover, he was often in intensive care where patients are sicker and risks are higher.

This is not to say you should stop or avoid the administration of IV fluids. But do be aware of the risks and, accordingly, monitor the hospital staff's maintenance on any line, be it a feeding tube, a drainage tube, a dialysis port, a catheter, or an IV access point.

What is IV line maintenance? It means cleaning and inspecting the site every day; redness may indicate infection. It means cleaning the lines regularly. It means changing the lines at certain intervals (or immediately if called for). Ask the hospital staff about their normal change-out frequency for IV lines. I was told that too-frequent changes actually increase the risk of infection. While that makes sense, I also noted that Bill only went septic from lines that were over three days old. So, once I knew the hospital's protocol, I always posted a sign indicating the date for Bill's next line change-out. If you can bear it, ask to watch while the nurse, doctor, or phlebotomist—a specially trained blood worker—inspects, cleans, and/or changes the line. If anything looks red, ask about it. If the offending line is removed promptly, you can often avoid problems.

Maintenance also means periodically moving the IV access points. The frequency varies with hospital protocol; I found that five days was the maximum for any single access point.

In some cases, generally more serious ones, an anesthesiologist may install a triple lumen, a device that provides access points for three separate lines. One of the three may be for liquid nutrition into the veins, as was the case for Bill until a feeding tube was inserted. Liquid nutrition increases the likelihood of line infection, so be extra vigilant in this case.

*Ask About Every Medication, Injection, and IV Solution*

Remember, though, that while IV lines are a route, the solutions they convey are worth your scrutiny and your questions, too. A rehabilitation worker told me about a close call while her father, a diabetic, was in the hospital and her mother was staying with him. One evening, a nurse brought a new IV solution into the room and began to hook up the tubing to her dad. When her mother casually asked what the new drug was, the nurse informed her it was D10W, a sugar solution.

What would have happened to her diabetic father had the question gone unasked and the sugar solution administered? Always ask about what will be flowing through those IV lines!

As a patient advocate, never hesitate to speak up. Better safe than sorry. Rosie O'Donnell once said, "Speak and you are criticized. Be silent and you are damned." Which would you prefer?

recommendation
9

# UNDERSTAND EVERY PROCEDURE *Used or Denied in Treatment*

USE THE FIVE W's to learn as much as you can from the doctors. Ask them (1) who? (2) what? (3) when? (4) where? and (5) why? And use some basic precautions to prevent spreading infection.

*No one is hurt by doing the right thing.*
—HAWAIIAN PROVERB

By now, the doctors and nurses should be accustomed to your participation in the care of your loved one. You've educated yourself. You ask plenty of questions about medicines, IV fluids, and other treatments. Now let's enhance our partnership by looking at medical procedures. But first, consider some important precautions.

## Precaution: Insist on Hand Washing

The single most important procedure for you and all care providers is scrupulous hand washing with soap and hot water. Dirty, non-sterile hands spread infection. Doctors making rounds can and do spread infection by failing to wash between rooms. You have a right and an obligation to insist that all healthcare workers wash their hands before and after seeing your patient. Improper hand washing by staff, visitors, and patients causes about one million of the two million annual cases of hospital-acquired infections, slightly less than half of which are fatal, according to the U.S. Centers for Disease Control and Prevention (CDC).[1]

Many hospital rooms have a dispenser with an alcohol-based sanitizer. Insist on soap-and-water hand washing anyway; these sanitizers only protect against one of the three top hospital-transmitted diseases described below.

There's a word for these hospital-acquired infections: nosocomial (nah-so-KOH-me-ul). There's also a word for diseases that are doctor-created: iatrogenic (eye-at-tro-GEN-ik). Unfortunately, these obscure words may help care providers obscure the truth of their role in spreading infection. Recall the words of the Hippocratic oath, "First, do no harm," and help your loved one's care providers live up to them.

1 HealthLink, "SARS? WNV? For Most, Common Infections Are the Real Worry," Medical College of Wisconsin, March 28, 2003, http://healthlink.mcw.edu/article/1031002230.html.

## Precaution: Know Some Common Hospital-Acquired Diseases

Let's look at three of the most common hospital-acquired diseases.

**MRSA** is the short name for multi-resistant staphylococcus aureus (STAFF-a-low-COK-us OR-ee-us). It is also called "methicillin-resistant." Both terms mean that the bacteria resist treatment—many antibiotics are ineffective with them. MRSA shows up most often as a skin infection, boil. or abscess, perhaps in a surgical wound or IV site. It may be swollen, red, and pus-filled. MRSA can spead, infecting the bones and joints. Especially when spread through central IV lines, MRSA can infect the bloodstream, a condition known as sepsis. In ICUs, this type of sepsis is the third most common kind of healthcare-associated infection, with an estimated 12 to 25 percent death rate.[2]



Symptoms include:

- high fever (possibly with low body temperature)
- fast breathing (hyperventilation)
- rapid heartbeat
- reddish skin rash
- decreased urine output
- organ failure
- confusion or delirium
- shaking
- warm skin[3]

When Bill went septic (thirteen times!), he had the first six symptoms listed above, but not all in every episode. With a hospital bill of about $25,000 per episode, Bill's sepsis added $300,000 to his total. At that rate, one would think

2 C. Muto, et al., "Reduction in Central Line–Associated Bloodstream Infections among Patients in Intensive Care Units—Pennsylvania, April 2001–March 2005," *Morbidity and Mortality Weekly Report*, Oct. 14, 2005.

3 eMedicineHealth, "Sepsis Symptoms," http://www.emedicinehealth.com/sepsis_blood_infection/page3_em.htm#Sepsis%20Symptoms.

hospitals would do anything to avoid this expense, not to mention the loss of life. But alas, it is not so in all cases.



**Nosocomial pneumonia** is also known as NP; it may also be called hospital-acquired, community-acquired, or ventilator-associated pneumonia (HAP, CAP, or VAP). It tends to be more serious than other types of pneumonia because the patient's ability to fight disease is already weakened, and hospitals contain more dangerous organisms than daily-life settings. The elderly, alcohol users, those with suppressed immune systems, and the recently ill are more susceptible to NP.[4]

Symptoms include:

- fever
- cough
- abnormal phlegm or mucous production
- malaise or "feeling lousy"
- fatigue
- difficulty breathing, or shortness of breath
- chest pain
- death

**Clostridium Difficile–Associated Disease** is also called CDAD or "C. diff." It is caused by the bacterium Clostridium difficile (kloh-STRIH-dee-um diff-ih-SEEL)—one of the "bad guys" in our gut. When the mix of good guys and bad guys gets out of balance and the C. diff bad guys go wild, typically after a course of antibiotics, a watery diarrhea results. C. diff causes about three million cases of diarrhea and colitis a year in the United States.[5] People with C. diff "shed spores in their stools that can be spread from person to person. Spores can survive up to

4 Health-Cares.net, "What Types of Pneumonia Are There?", http://respiratory-lung.health-cares.net/pneumonia-types.php.

5 Bryan Tungland, "Dreamfields Pasta: A Healthy Meal Addition for Clostridium difficile: A Reoccurring Problem in Hospitals and Nursing Homes," Dreamfields Foods, http://dreamfieldsfoods.com/downloads/Clostridium_difficile.pdf.

70 days in the environment and can be transported on the hands of healthcare personnel who have direct contact with infected patients or with environmental surfaces (floors, bedpans, toilets, telephones, stethoscopes, etc.) contaminated with C. difficile."[6] Symptoms include watery diarrhea, crampy abdominal pain, abdominal tenderness, fever, and pus or blood in the diarrhea.[7]

A University of Minnesota Medical School study showed that in U.S. hospitals, rates of colitis caused by this bacteria "jumped 109 percent between 1993 and 2003 . . . C. difficile colitis became more severe over that time period and caused more deaths among hospital patients."[8]

---

Hospital-acquired infections involve many risk factors, including hospital procedures, personnel, and buildings, as well the severity of the original illness.[9] We can hope that hospitals minimize the risks, but we have no control over these efforts. What can we do? We can:

- wash our hands meticulously before we enter a room
- put on a gown, mask, and/or gloves before we enter a room
- discourage people who are ill from visiting our patient
- wash our hands again when we leave the room

We can also insist that all healthcare staff wash their hands before and after treating or examining our patient. Have I made my point?

---

6 Ibid.

7 InteliHealth, "Antibiotic-Associated Diarrhea," Mar. 28, 2007, http://www.intelihealth.com/IH/ihtIH/WSIHW000/9339/9468.html#symptoms.

8 JAMA/Archives Journals, "Bacterial Colitis on the Rise in U.S. Hospitals," *HealthDay News*, July 17, 2007, http://healthfinder.gov/news/newsstory.asp?docID=606415.

9 Quoc V. Nguyen, "Hospital-Acquired Infections," eMedicine from WebMD, http://www.emedicine.com/ped/topic1619.htm.

## Procedures: Use the Five W's

In journalism, reporters learn to use the Five W's. Let's put them to use, triggering relevant questions for us to ask about any procedure planned for our loved one.

9

*Understand Every Procedure Used or Denied in Treatment*

- Who? What? When? Where? Why? (and often "How?")

Whenever a procedure is planned, it suggests that a change is underway or is anticipated. In general, to deal with change, people need to know:

- Where are we going?
- Why is this necessary?
- How will we get there?
- Who is involved, and what part will everyone play in getting us there?

In a larger sense, there's another "W" here: WE. We are a team. The patient, the doctor, and the patient advocate form a powerful triangle. This is not a case of doctor decides, patient complies. This is a case of WE. If the doctor ignores any part of the WE, there is no triangle. And what happens when one leg of a tripod is removed? Make sure you are personally involved in every procedure that affects your loved one.

Ask the doctor all the questions listed below. In addition to the answers themselves, look for eye contact, cautiousness, candor, and compassion. Ask any questions that will help you determine what you, as an advocate, can do to improve the odds in favor of your patient.

- ***Who—***
  - ✓ Who should be involved in this procedure?
  - ✓ Who will be involved in this procedure?
  - ✓ Who will not be involved?
  - ✓ Who will play each role?
  - ✓ Who will actually perform the procedure?

✓ Who will keep you informed during the procedure?

✓ Who will care for the patient afterward?

If you know the players and the roles they will play, you have a far better chance of gaining their commitment and ensuring their readiness. Sometimes, due to staffing, illness, or other variables, the best possible medical partner is not available on the day the procedure is scheduled. Does it make sense to delay it? Is there greater risk in the delay, or in going with a second-choice partner?



- **What—**

✓ What is going to happen?

✓ What could happen?

✓ What alternatives have been or could be considered?

✓ What has the physician done to lower the risk of complications?

✓ What can you as advocate do, before, during, and after the procedure?

✓ What will the outcome look like?

✓ What will it feel like for your loved one, the patient?

✓ What would the physician do if he/she were in the patient's position?

The "what" of the discussion helps us know the road. It's like being given a map or a compass and told how to read it. Confidence in the outcome increases when we know the direction, where the detours exist and how long the trip will last.

- **When—**

✓ When should the procedure take place?

✓ When will the procedure take place? (If a delay is indicated, perhaps because of hospital variables, what are the consequences of delay? Do they outweigh the benefits of waiting?)

✓ When can you expect to see your loved one after the procedure?

- **Where—**
  - ✓ Where is the best place for the procedure to be performed?
  - ✓ Where will the procedure be performed? (If any location factors indicate a delay, what are the consequences of delay? Do they outweigh the benefits of waiting?)
- **Why—**
  - ✓ Why are we doing this?

### *Checklist F: Procedure Preparation*

| NUMBER | QUESTIONS TO ASK | ✓ |
|---|---|---|
| **1.** | **Who—** | |
| a. | Who *should* be involved in this procedure? | |
| b. | Who *will* be involved in this procedure? | |
| c. | Who will not be involved? | |
| d. | Who will play each role? | |
| e. | Who will actually perform the procedure? | |
| f. | Who will keep you informed during the procedure? | |
| g. | Who will care for your family member after the procedure? | |
| **2.** | **What—** | |
| a. | What is going to happen? | |
| b. | What could happen? | |
| c. | What alternatives have been or could be considered? | |
| d. | What has the physician done to lower the risk of complications? | |
| e. | What can you, as advocate, do before, during, and after the procedure? | |
| f. | What will the outcome look like? | |
| g. | What is it going to feel like for your loved one, the patient? | |
| h. | What would the physician do if a member of his/her own family were in the patient's position? | |
| **3.** | **When—** | |
| a. | When *should* the procedure take place? | |
| b. | When *will* the procedure take place? (If a delay is indicated, perhaps because of hospital variables, what are the consequences of delay? Do they outweigh the benefits of waiting?) | |
| c. | When can you expect to see your loved one after the procedure? | |

*Understand Every Procedure Used or Denied in Treatment*

*Continued on next page*

*Checklist F (continued)*

9

Understand Every Procedure Used or Denied in Treatment

| NUMBER | QUESTIONS TO ASK | ✓ |
|---|---|---|
| 4. | **Where:** | |
| a. | Where is the best place for this procedure to be performed? | |
| b. | Where *will* the procedure take place? (If any location factors indicate a delay, what are the consequences of delay? Do they outweigh the benefits of waiting?) | |
| 5. | **Why—** | |
| a. | Why are we doing this? | |

*recommendation* 10

# KEEP TRACK OF ALL SUPPLIES AND SERVICES, *Warranted and Unwarranted*

Refuse to pay for duplicate or unnecessary supplies and services. As you accumulate supplies, post signs in the hospital room for staff to look in specified drawers/places for usable supplies.

*Learn the rules so you know how to break them properly.*
—Nepalese Good Luck Mantra

*Keep Track of All Supplies and Services, Warranted and Unwarranted*

When Bill left the hospital, he owned fourteen blood pressure cuffs and three pairs of $600 inflatable boots (to prevent blood clots). Other duplications were equally excessive—and preventable, if only his nurse had checked to see if we already had an item before she entered the room with it in hand. And, because Bill had MRSA (a contagious staph infection), once an item was in the room, we owned it! Even after posting a sign—"Please do not order or deliver new supplies to this room without first checking the bedside nightstand"—I could not stop the inflow.

So my recommendation here is brief: post such a sign in your loved one's room, then inform the hospital that it is there and that you will not pay for duplicate supplies. Then, if it happens, ask that the charge be removed from your record—and insist on seeing it removed, even if the reaction is testy. Often I was promised that a charge would be removed, only to have it appear on my bill. Once it gets there it is virtually immovable, so you must act upstream from this event.

The same goes for doctor consultations that are not requested and are not warranted. For example, because I was present in Bill's room 24/7, I was there when a plastic surgeon arrived to assess Bill for the need for plastic surgery. Guess what part of Bill's body he inspected? His butt! Yes, a plastic surgeon assessed the need for cosmetic treatment at the site of Bill's bedsore. I contested the need for this consult, the doctor agreed, and we managed to have it removed from the bill. This should not happen, but it does!

Remember, every duplicated or unnecessary dollar removed from your bill is a dollar that stays available within your insurance policy's lifetime maximum. It is a dollar that can be used for what it is intended to provide: healthcare.

recommendation
II

# ARRANGE FOR *24/7 Coverage*

THAT'S TWENTY-FOUR HOURS a day, seven days a week. You are the guardian, so maintain your post or pass it to someone else. This is especially true in intensive care.

*The greatest gift you can give another is the purity of your attention.*
—RICHARD MOSS,
*The I That Is We*

11

*Arrange for 24/7 Coverage*

Patient advocacy is a full-time job. I recommend that you arrange for 24/7 coverage for your loved one. Form an educated, consistent "care team" consisting of yourself and a few trusted others. Round-the-clock presence is key, with the advocate either sleeping in the patient's room or nearby, depending on hospital policy.

Bill and I were lucky. I am self-employed, and I was able to shut down my consulting practice to be at his side day and night—without losing my client base. We were lucky to have great health insurance, otherwise our astronomical medical bills would have driven us to bankruptcy. We were lucky to both have disability insurance, otherwise we would have suffered, at a minimum, extreme financial hardship. We were also very fortunate to have the loyal support of friends and family. Without exception, all stood with us through the most difficult time of our lives. They continue to support us to this day.

Draw on your own support network for your care team. It helps for one of you—probably you, if you are reading this book—to serve as the primary advocate, the organizer and information clearinghouse. Consider these sources for other members of your care team:

- family
- friends
- members of your faith community
- work colleagues
- neighbors
- parents of children's friends
- school-related acquaintances
- social organization members
- local volunteer agencies (especially for transportation and meal delivery)

As you form your team, try to anticipate the times when the patient will be most vulnerable. You may want to cover them yourself, or ask for especially close monitoring at those times, when things are more likely to go wrong. These might include eating, bathing, exercising, being transferred from place to place, or undergoing a procedure such as an X ray, among other things. Even physical therapy has its risks. I knew a man who died one day before his discharge date: while he was doing physical therapy in the gym, the nurse monitoring him stepped away for five minutes, during which he suffered a fatal heart attack.

To stay organized and in touch with each other, create a Care Team Notebook. Prepare it before your loved one's admission, or soon thereafter, if the stay is expected to last more than one overnight. And when people ask, "What can I do?" the notebook can offer some ideas.

*Arrange for 24/7 Coverage*

Divide a three-ring binder into several sections (ideally with tabs and/or different paper colors); see the samples that follow this section.

- **Sign-up Sheets.** Let members choose their "on-duty" shifts. Make sign-up sheets divided into shifts of at least four hours. (Note: Find out what times your hospital's staff has their own shift change, and make sure yours do *not* fall at the same time. These are vulnerable times for your patient, and an advocate can help provide continuity.)
- **Doctor Visits.** On these sheets, care team members record every doctor visit, and its outcome, occurring during their shift.
- **Procedures.** Record any procedures done, expected outcome, and actual outcome.
- **Notes.** Write down any noteworthy observations.
- **Questions.** List any questions to be asked of medical personnel in future shifts.
- **Outside-the-Hospital Tasks and Chores.** This is a sign-up sheet for tasks to help keep your family and household functioning. Categorize tasks such as child care, household chores, transportation, patient's personal needs, and so on.
- **Legal Documents.** For reference, include a copy of the Durable Medical Power of Attorney and the living will; and other relevant documents.
- **Emergency Contact Information.** Include information for yourself as well as key medical personnel.

Sample forms follow here, as well as a suggested introduction for the notebook. They can also be found at www.hospitalstayhandbook.com.

To keep family and friends updated on your loved one's condition, consider caringbridge.com. This free service lets you create a blog—an updatable "Web log" with its own Internet address. You can easily update it with information about the patient, other comments, thoughts, and requests, and expressions of gratitude, and perhaps even your "care team" needs. With these postings, you need not personally contact everyone in your network when there is news. And those people who crave information can get it without worrying about bothering the family. (I wish I had known of this tool during Bill's illness.)

The most important way in which Bill and I were lucky was this: he survived. But luck was only one factor: I believe my 24/7 vigil played a critical role in preventing this loss. So be ready for round-the-clock presence with the help of your care team. With your vigilance comes the certainty that you need never second-guess yourself: you are doing all you can on behalf of your loved one.

## Care Team Notebook Introduction

I am so grateful that you have expressed an interest in helping [*name of patient*] through this trying time. Each of you brings certain gifts and preferences and we appreciate any assistance you can provide, both in the hospital and otherwise. Our most pressing need is to find care team members so [*name of patient*] can have 24/7 support. As a team member, you would offer companionship and support as needed, monitor the patient's care, and record in writing any information about doctor visits, medical procedures, general notes, and questions that need to be raised (see numbers 2–5 below). Additionally, we need help at home (see number 6).

This book represents the "central repository" of activities. It has eight sections.

1. **Sign-Up Sheets.** Choose your "on-duty" four-hour shifts here. Together, we plan to provide round-the-clock coverage. We are especially thankful for night and weekend monitoring. Medical mistakes are the seventh-leading cause of death in the United States, and we don't want to become a statistic!
2. **Doctor Visit Records.** On these sheets, record every doctor visit during your shift, and the outcome of that visit.
3. **Medical Procedure Records.** Here, record any procedures done, the expected outcome, and the actual outcome.
4. **Notes.** Here, record any general observations about the patient, staff, or anything that seems noteworthy.
5. **Questions.** Here, list any questions to be asked of staff in a future shift.
6. **Outside-the-Hospital Tasks and Chores.** Sign up here to help us with other tasks: patient's personal needs, childcare, transportation, home chores, and so on.
7. **Legal Documents.** For your reference, here are copies of the Durable Medical Power of Attorney, the living will, and other relevant documents.
8. **Emergency Contact Information** for the family and key medical personnel.

Please review what we need and if you are willing and able to help, indicate where and when on the sign-up sheet(s). Thanks again for your support!

________________________________________

*(Your Signature)*

## Care Team Sign-Up Sheet

| DATE: | |
|---|---|
| **Hours of Shift** | **Care Team member** |
| 6 AM–10 AM | |
| 10 AM–2 PM | |
| 2 PM–6 PM | |
| 6 PM–10 PM | |
| 10 PM–2 AM | |
| 2 AM–6 AM | |

| DATE: | |
|---|---|
| **Hours of Shift** | **Care Team member** |
| 6 AM–10 AM | |
| 10 AM–2 PM | |
| 2 PM–6 PM | |
| 6 PM–10 PM | |
| 10 PM–2 AM | |
| 2 AM–6 AM | |

| DATE: | |
|---|---|
| **Hours of Shift** | **Care Team member** |
| 6 AM–10 AM | |
| 10 AM–2 PM | |
| 2 PM–6 PM | |
| 6 PM–10 PM | |
| 10 PM–2 AM | |
| 2 AM–6 AM | |

## Doctor Visits

Care team: Please record all doctor visits as shown below.

| DATE: | | | | |
|---|---|---|---|---|
| Shift | Dr. Name | Service | Notes | Care Team Signature |
| 6 AM–10 AM | | | | |
| 10 AM–2 PM | | | | |
| 2 PM–6 PM | | | | |
| 6 PM–10 PM | | | | |
| 10 PM–2 AM | | | | |
| 2 AM–6 AM | | | | |

| DATE: | | | | |
|---|---|---|---|---|
| Shift | Dr. Name | Service | Notes | Care Team Signature |
| 6 AM–10 AM | | | | |
| 10 AM–2 PM | | | | |
| 2 PM–6 PM | | | | |
| 6 PM–10 PM | | | | |
| 10 PM–2 AM | | | | |
| 2 AM–6 AM | | | | |

## Medical Procedures

Care team: Please record details of all medical procedure as shown below.

| DATE: | | | | |
|---|---|---|---|---|
| **Shift** | **Dr. Name** | **Procedure** | **Expected Outcome** | **Actual Outcome** |
| 6 AM–10 AM | | | | |
| 10 AM–2 PM | | | | |
| 2 PM–6 PM | | | | |
| 6 PM–10 PM | | | | |
| 10 PM–2 AM | | | | |
| 2 AM–6 AM | | | | |

| DATE: | | | | |
|---|---|---|---|---|
| **Shift** | **Dr. Name** | **Procedure** | **Expected Outcome** | **Actual Outcome** |
| 6 AM–10 AM | | | | |
| 10 AM–2 PM | | | | |
| 2 PM–6 PM | | | | |
| 6 PM–10 PM | | | | |
| 10 PM–2 AM | | | | |
| 2 AM–6 AM | | | | |

## Notes

Care team: Write down any relevant observations about the patient, staff, or anything noteworthy.

| DATE: | | | |
|---|---|---|---|
| **Shift** | **Observation** | **What do you think caused this?** | **CT Signature** |
| 6 AM–10 AM | | | |
| 10 AM–2 PM | | | |
| 2 PM–6 PM | | | |
| 6 PM–10 PM | | | |
| 10 PM–2 AM | | | |
| 2 AM–6 AM | | | |

| DATE: | | | |
|---|---|---|---|
| **Shift** | **Observation** | **What do you think caused this?** | **CT Signature** |
| 6 AM–10 AM | | | |
| 10 AM–2 PM | | | |
| 2 PM–6 PM | | | |
| 6 PM–10 PM | | | |
| 10 PM–2 AM | | | |
| 2 AM–6 AM | | | |

## Questions

Care team: Write down any questions that need to be asked during a future shift.

| DATE: | | | |
|---|---|---|---|
| **Shift** | **Question** | **Why are you asking this?** | **CT Signature** |
| 6 AM–10 AM | | | |
| 10 AM–2 PM | | | |
| 2 PM–6 PM | | | |
| 6 PM–10 PM | | | |
| 10 PM–2 AM | | | |
| 2 AM–6 AM | | | |

| DATE: | | | |
|---|---|---|---|
| **Shift** | **Question** | **Why are you asking this?** | **CT Signature** |
| 6 AM–10 AM | | | |
| 10 AM–2 PM | | | |
| 2 PM–6 PM | | | |
| 6 PM–10 PM | | | |
| 10 PM–2 AM | | | |
| 2 AM–6 AM | | | |

## Outside-the-Hospital Tasks Sign-Up Sheets

| Category | Task | Care Team Member |
|---|---|---|
| **Personal care for patient** | | |
| | | |
| | | |
| **Child care / Elder care** | | |
| | | |
| | | |
| **Transportation** | | |
| | | |
| | | |
| **Household chores** | | |
| | | |
| | | |

## Legal Documents

(please return originals to this notebook)

## Emergency Contact Information

| Name | Preferred Contact Number | Alternative Contact Number |
|---|---|---|
| Spouse/Significant Other: | | |
| Adult Child: | | |
| Adult Child: | | |
| Spiritual Adviser: | | |
| Doctor: | | |
| Doctor: | | |
| Doctor: | | |
| Friend: | | |
| Friend: | | |
| Neighbor: | | |
| | | |
| | | |

recommendation
12

# PRAY

*Believe more deeply. Hold your face up to the light, even though for the moment you do not see.*

—Bill Wilson, cofounder of Alcoholics Anonymous

I strongly believe in the power of prayer—one's own prayers, and those of others. In fact, documented studies show that patients who are prayed for have a greater probability of survival. Although the "why" of these results cannot be explained, the results speak for themselves.

How we pray and to whom is our personal choice. Embrace your own belief system and practice what it tells you. For me, prayer is intention. When I state and hold an intention that is for the greater good, I am in prayer. For some of us, prayer means a bended knee, a bowed head or a lifted head, or perhaps facing a certain direction. For some it means dance, for some, meditation.

Prayer does not have to be directed to "God as we understand Him," in the words of the Twelve-Step approach. In fact, some newcomers to Alcoholics Anonymous turn to their meeting group as their Higher Power, particularly if they have lost their own belief system and not yet rediscovered it. Prayer is a concept that can be held inside both religion and spirituality. Whether you actively practice a religion, are agnostic, or define your belief system as "spirituality," prayer can find a home with you.

I think of prayer as communion with something bigger than myself. And in my case, only something far bigger than myself could hold all the pain, fear, and anger associated with my journey through the healthcare system.

This is not the time to question your belief, but rather to embrace it and ask for help. The goal you seek, however, cannot be the miracle of survival itself, for we do not hold another's life in our hands. We hold another's life in our heart, with our love. The hands that hold all life are bigger than ours . . .

The renowned shaman Sandra Ingerman has said:

> All miracles involve union with a divine force. In the Bible, when Jesus says to "heal in my name," the true Aramaic translation of this is "to know God and heal as God does." This means to have union with the creative force of life is essential for true healing to take place. Sai Baba, a guru in India, is known for his miraculous acts and healing abilities. He says, "The only difference between me and you is I know who I am and you don't" (meaning he knows he is divine). Love is an essential ingredient in all miracles as it is only love that heals.

> Techniques don't heal. Where there is an open heart there is the energy to bring through miraculous and magical energy. Love is the great transformer.[1]

In our case, people all over the world prayed for Bill. Closer to home, the church across the street from our house included him in a weekly prayer circle, thanks to one of its members, a colleague of Bill's. Every week the leader of the circle called me for an update: "What body part should we pray for this time?" I saw a direct correlation between their prayers and the sequence of Bill's gradual healing. His kidneys started functioning after weeks of prayer focus. Later, his feeding tube came out and he began to eat following a similar focus. Gratitude came in big gulps of air for me and food for Bill.



If you need to know more about your faith, contact your minister, rabbi, priest, teacher, imam, reverend, elder, shaman, holy man or woman, or church leader. Be very clear about what you want, and do not hesitate to ask for it in prayer. You have nothing to lose and everything to gain. So does your loved one, whatever the outcome. You will know then that you have done everything that could be done. You can let go and surrender.

---

1 Sandra Ingerman, *Medicine for the Earth: How to Transform Personal and Environmental Toxins* (New York: Three Rivers Press, 2000).

*recommendation*
13

# SURRENDER

*Have patience with everything unresolved in your heart*
*and try to love the questions themselves . . .*
*Don't search for the answers,*
*which could not be given to you now,*
*because you would not be able to live them.*
—Rainer Maria Rilke

There is nothing like a serious illness to remind us how powerless we are. Those in Twelve-Step recovery programs phrase their First Step this way: ". . . made a decision to turn my will and my life over to the care of God, as I understood Him."[1] This is surrender. You are responsible for the input. You are not responsible for the outcome.

According to Rich Work's book *Awaken to the Healer Within*, certain universal laws govern all creation. In Recommendation 6, "Assume Your Loved One Can Hear Everything," we looked at two of them, the Law of Magnetic Attraction and the Law of Creative Manifestation. Here is a third:

> ***The Law of Allowing***
> This is the most difficult law of all. Put your thoughts into universal consciousness, reinforced by desire. Then step aside and allow the universe to manifest it for you. If you are hoping, then you are not allowing. If you have expectations, you are not allowing.
>
> If you have expectations, it is like saying, "Okay, God, this is what I want. Now, let me tell you how to do it!" And God responds by saying, "For heaven's sake, get out of the way and let me do it for you." The more you expect, the more you hope, the more you try to manage or control, the more you will interfere and retard the manifesting of your desires. The Law of Allowing means just that. After all, the Master said, "Ask and ye shall receive." He didn't say, "ask and we'll go have a committee meeting and take a vote on it."[2]

If you have done everything discussed in the previous chapters, you have done everything you can. It is time to surrender, to let go. Sometimes we need help understanding how and when to surrender. The most helpful guidance I have found on this subject is in the book *Managing Personal Change* by C. D. Scott and D. T. Jaffe.[3] This book includes a grid that helps us determine an appropriate response to any given situation.

---

1 *Alcoholics Anonymous,* 4th ed. (New York: AA World Services, Inc., 2001), 59.

2 Rich Work with Ann Marie Groth, *Awaken to the Healer Within*, 23–24.

3 C. D. Scott and D. T. Jaffe, *Managing Personal Change: Self Management Skills for Work and Life Transitions* (Los Altos, CA: Crisp Publications, 1989).

**Personal Power—Getting What You Want**

| | *CAN CONTROL* | *CANNOT CONTROL* |
|---|---|---|
| *TAKE ACTION* | Mastery<br>*achievement & success* | Ceaseless Striving<br>*frustration & anger* |
| *NO ACTION* | Giving Up<br>*helpless & hopeless* | Letting Go<br>*relief & release* |



Here's what this means. In life, the authors point out, there are some things you *can* control and some things you *cannot* control. Recognizing this will help you understand whether you should try to take action.

When you can control something—such as how you behave, how you treat healthcare providers, how you respond to crises, and how you learn new medical information—you should take action. This will give you feelings of achievement and success, say the authors. For example, I learned everything I could about Bill's disease, treatment, medications, procedures, and prognosis, and was successful in many of my efforts.

On the other hand, if you can't control something, don't keep trying. If you "ceaselessly strive" to do something that is beyond your control, you end up frustrated and angry. In fact, you can test the difference between what you *can* and *cannot* control that way. If you feel frustrated and angry, you are probably trying to do something that is beyond your control. That sounds like me when I ceaselessly strove to make the doctors at Hospital B do what I wanted them to do. When I finally complained about it to the Patient Rights advocate, I moved back into mastery, and then into letting go.

If you can't control it, just as you can't control whether your loved one lives or dies, let go: find the relief and release of admitting it is out of your control. Then put your energies elsewhere—such as into mastering what you can control.

But if you can control it, don't fail to take action. That would be giving up. If you are feeling helpless and hopeless, that's a good indicator you have given up when you could be doing something for your loved one or yourself. You want to be in mastery and in letting go. Over nearly eight months, only Hospital B gave up on Bill.

If you add your voice to mastery, by a Native American definition of leadership, you cannot be ignored. According to a Native American tradition, true leaders (advocates) have "three kinds of power": first, presence, or charisma; second, communication skills; and third, position, that is, a committed opinion about a subject. "The presence of all three indicates 'big personal power' and you cannot be ignored!"[4]

By now, the healthcare providers cannot ignore you! Feel good about what you have done for your loved one, and keep on doing it. But remember, we cannot control life and death—our own or another's. There is a higher order of things at work in the universe.

Sometimes letting go is an active process because, in order to make a decision of that magnitude, you have to set aside your own desire to keep your loved one with you. At some point, you and your healthcare partners may come to the conclusion that the quality of life remaining for your loved one is poor. If a "do not resuscitate" order is in place, it may be that your loved one will pass peacefully on his/her own. In the absence of such direction, you may be left with an excruciating decision—what medical intervention will I allow in maintaining the life of my loved one? This is a very personal decision and one that must be made with great care and compassion. It is often helpful to involve others in the decision-making process, not only physicians but non-physician mediators such as hospital staff ethicists, patient advocates, social workers, and clergy members. Once values are explicitly discussed and differences clarified, a plan may be agreed upon by which all parties can abide.

4 Angeles Arrien, *The Four-Fold Way.*

*recommendation*
14

# TAKE CARE *of Yourself*

You are of no value to your loved one if you go down for the count. Sacrificing your own health for another is not what anyone who loves you would want you to do. "Take care of yourself" is my first and last recommendation to you, because all the others depend on it.

*If you are not good for yourself,*
*how can you be good for another?*
—Spanish Proverb

The Alzheimer's Association has identified "Ten Warning Signs of Caregiver Stress" and has generously granted permission to reprint them here.[1] I offer them now as a final caution, with my own commentary. Use them to prevent needing an advocate yourself because *you* end up in the hospital!



**TEN WARNING SIGNS OF CAREGIVER STRESS**

1. DENIAL about the disease and its effects on the person who has been diagnosed.
2. ANGER at the person who is sick or others. Anger about the treatments. Anger that people don't understand what is going on.
3. SOCIAL WITHDRAWAL from friends and activities that once brought pleasure.
4. ANXIETY about facing another day and what the future holds.
5. DEPRESSION begins to break your spirit and affects your ability to cope.
6. EXHAUSTION makes it nearly impossible to complete necessary daily tasks.
7. SLEEPLESSNESS caused by a never-ending list of concerns.
8. IRRITABILITY leads to moodiness and triggers negative responses and reactions.
9. LACK OF CONCENTRATION makes it difficult to perform familiar tasks.
10. HEALTH PROBLEMS begin to take their toll, both mentally and physically.

### *1. DENIAL about the disease and its effects on the person who has been diagnosed.*

Denial could also make us believe that the hospital will care for our loved ones with the same attention and love that we ourselves can provide.

---

1 Alzheimer Society of Canada, "Caring for Someone with Alzheimer's Disease? Take Care of Yourself Too!", Alzheimer Care: Caregiver Support, 1995, http://www.alzheimer.ca/english/care/caregivers-selfcare.htm. Reprinted with permission.

***2. ANGER at the person who is sick or others. Anger about the treatments. Anger that people don't understand what is going on.***

Although I never got angry at Bill, I did get very angry at the hospital staff on occasion, and my anger did not help resolve the issues.

***3. SOCIAL WITHDRAWAL from friends and activities that once brought pleasure.***

Both at the hospital and later at home, I was so tired that if my friends had not come to me, I would not have asked them to do so. And yet, it is these very people and the cherished activities of my free time that refresh and revitalize me.

***4. ANXIETY about facing another day and what the future holds.***

Constant vigilance is wearying. At the hospital I often wondered if anything else could go wrong! Sometimes I still do.

***5. DEPRESSION begins to break your spirit and affects your ability to cope.***

Watch out for this sneaky feeling! It creeps up with little to no warning. Because it is so gradual, it is often hard to identify and, for some of us (like me), hard to own.

***6. EXHAUSTION makes it nearly impossible to complete necessary daily tasks.***

We frequently hear the term "double-digit inflation" from our politicians. Well, I can beat that! I had quintuple-digit sleep loss!

***7. SLEEPLESSNESS caused by a never-ending list of concerns.***

Talk about lists! In the hospital, there were lists of compromised body parts, lists of medication interactions to watch for, lists of supplies, lists of nurses' names, lists of doctors' names and on and on and on! You are only one person, even if you are superhuman!

*8. IRRITABILITY leads to moodiness and triggers negative responses and reactions.*

In fairness, I must admit that, on *rare* occasions, I *may* have overreacted just a tiny bit. And I'm sure some of Bill's healthcare providers would agree.



*9. LACK OF CONCENTRATION makes it difficult to perform familiar tasks.*

Even after seven and a half months in the hospital, I would sometimes find myself walking down the hall to the nurses' station, unable to recall the purpose of my trip.

*10. HEALTH PROBLEMS begin to take their toll, both mentally and physically.*

I ended up at the foot doctor with heel pain because of all the walking I had done at the hospital and later at home. I also found myself in psychotherapy, learning how to deal with my personal losses as well as the "new man" in my life: Bill.

---

Neither you nor your loved one can go through a life-changing event such as a serious extended illness without having your lives change. That is true for both Bill and me. Bill is in therapy to deal with his personal losses as well as the "new woman" in his life: me. Because we are different, because we have both experienced loss, and because we have discovered that life cannot be controlled, we are slowly learning that life can only be lived. This continues to be a hard lesson.

Assuming you have been taking care of yourself throughout this process, hope is the last piece of the puzzle. As so eloquently stated by Emily Dickinson, "Hope is the thing with feathers / That perches in the soul / And sings the tune without the words / And never stops at all."[2] Ask for help, if you need help to hope.

2 Emily Dickinson, "Hope Is the Thing with Feathers," *Complete Poems* (Boston: Little, Brown, 1924).

No matter what the outcome, time will help. We had to wait three months for Bill's pseudocysts to "ripen." We had to wait five months following surgery for Bill's discharge. Bill continues to wait for an explanation of what he is to do with the rest of his life. I had to wait six months before the pain of our experience had eased enough that I could write this book.

And, no matter what the outcome is, whatever you did was the best you could do, and the rest is out of your hands. Spending time "should-ing" on yourself does not help recovery. It only prolongs it. Be gentle, love yourself, and trust this process. Know that even as a stranger, I am very proud that you did what you could. I am also grateful if I played some small role in assisting you.

We started this journey together with a reminder that we do this for love. And we did. May you walk hand in hand with your loved one through all eternity.

# FOR A DEEPER UNDERSTANDING

# LESSONS IN ADVOCACY

*One of the most important steps you can take to help calm the storm is to not allow yourself to be taken in a flurry of overwrought emotion or desperation thereby accidentally contributing to the swale and the swirl.*

—Clarissa Pinkola Estés

Imagine yourself in the role of patient for a moment. When we are ill or injured, we are not at our best. We may be dealing with pain, loss, fear, and many other issues—physical and emotional background noises that make it hard for us to hear what is said, much less attend to that which is not spoken. Not only that, but consider our physical position: we're often horizontal, on our back. No wonder it's especially hard to ask questions, challenge decisions, and try to partner with our doctor. That doctor is probably:

- leaning over us from a standing position, fully clothed
- placing cold objects such as stethoscopes onto our nude body
- probing or pushing on the part of our body giving us the greatest discomfort
- poking us with sharp objects
- speaking to us as if we were a condition or body part; perhaps discussing us as if we weren't in the room

In this disadvantaged position, wouldn't we do better if another person or persons stepped forward on our behalf?

## Your Work as an Advocate



That is the role of the advocate. If you are reading this book, that is probably the role you are assuming. Advocacy is sacred work, and we cannot depend on others to do it for us, especially those who work within the healthcare community. It requires a connection to our self, our patient, our families and friends, the healthcare community, our spiritual beliefs, and the universe. Many of us don't understand this need for connection; we don't know how to expand our world in the midst of a medical crisis.

As broken as the U.S. healthcare system is today, those who work within it cannot change it from the inside. If they could, wouldn't they have done it by now? That leaves this work to us, and we must be prepared to fight for partnership with healthcare providers—because our patient's life may ultimately depend on it. It is time for the partnership model to emerge. You can and should be an equal member of the healthcare team!

You will be expected to be fully present in every exchange, every decision, every negotiation on the patient's behalf. This is your work as an advocate. Your emotions will be activated, and you will be expected to bring your body, mind, and spirit into this work. You cannot hold another's life in your hands and remain disengaged.

Having said this, let me remind you of the importance of detachment. Harrison Owen offers these Four Immutable Laws of the Spirit, which guide every negotiation and every life on this planet:

1. Whoever shows up are exactly the right people.
2. When it happens, it's always the right time.
3. Whatever happens is the only thing that can happen.
4. When it's over, it's over.[1]

1 Angeles Arrien, *Change, Conflict, and Resolution from a Cross-Cultural Perspective*, 4 audiocassettes read by the author (Petaluma, CA: Arrien Books & Tapes, n.d.).

Therefore, if you are here, you are exactly the right person at exactly the right time! In the words of former Czech president Václav Havel:

> I feel that the dormant goodwill in people needs to be stirred. People need to hear that it makes sense to behave decently or to help others, to place common interests above their own, to respect the elementary rules of human coexistence . . . people want to hear that decency and courage make sense, that something must be risked in the struggle . . . They want to know that they are not alone, forgotten, written off.[2]



The following introduction to patient advocacy is addressed to the patient. It is reprinted here with permission from the National Patient Safety Foundation.

2 Václav Havel, *Summer Meditations* (New York: Vintage, 1993).

## NATIONAL PATIENT SAFETY FOUNDATION® (NPSF)
### A Consumer Fact Sheet: The Role of the Patient Advocate



*Illness is a stressful time for patients as well as for their families. The best laid plans can go awry, judgment is impaired, and put simply, you are not at your best when you are sick. Patients need someone who can look out for their best interests and help navigate the confusing healthcare system–in other words, an advocate.*

What is a patient advocate? An advocate is a "supporter, believer, sponsor, promoter, campaigner, backer, or spokesperson." It is important to consider all of these aspects when choosing an advocate for yourself or someone in your family. An effective advocate is someone you trust who is willing to act on your behalf as well as someone who can work well with other members of your healthcare team such as your doctors and nurses.

An advocate may be a member of your family, such as a spouse, a child, another family member, or a close friend. Another type of advocate is a professional advocate. Hospitals usually have professionals who play this role called patient representatives or patient advocates. Social workers, nurses, and chaplains may also fill this role. These advocates can often be very helpful in cutting through red tape. It is helpful to find out if your hospital has professional advocates available, and how they may be able to help you.

### *Using an advocate–Getting started*

1. Select a person you can communicate with and you trust. It's important to pick someone who is assertive and who has good communication skills. Make sure the person you select is willing and able to be the type of advocate you need.
2. Decide what you want help with and what you want to handle on your own. For example, you may want help with:
   a. clarifying your options for hospitals, doctors, diagnostic tests and procedures or treatment choices
   b. getting information or asking specific questions

c. writing down information you receive from your caregivers, as well as any questions you may have

d. assuring your wishes are carried out when you may not be able to do that by yourself.

3. Decide if you would like your advocate to accompany you to tests, appointments, treatments and procedures. If so, insist your doctor and other caregivers allow this.



4. Be very clear with your advocate about what you would like them to know and be involved in:

   a. treatment decisions?

   b. any change in your condition?

   c. test results?

   d. keeping track of medications?

5. Let your physician and those caring for you know who your advocate is and how you want them involved in your care.

6. Arrange for your designated advocate to be the spokesperson for the rest of your family and make sure your other family members know this. This will provide a consistent communication link for your caregivers and can help to minimize confusion and misunderstandings within your family. Make sure your doctor and nurses have your advocate's phone number and make sure your advocate has the numbers for your providers, hospital and pharmacy, as well as anyone else you may want to contact in the case of an emergency.

### *Patient safety suggestions–Getting started*

1. Ask questions, read labels, ask for explanations; take nothing for granted.

2. Ask for written information about medications you are given in the hospital and when you go home.

3. Don't be afraid to question something you don't understand.

4. Insist that staff check your armband before they take you for tests, give you oral medications or put anything in your intravenous fluids.
5. Pay attention to your symptoms—pain, nausea, drowsiness, dizziness. Often these are side effects of medications or treatments. Don't ignore them. Make sure your doctors and nurses know how you are feeling.
6. Always ask for help if something just doesn't "feel right."
7. Ask *what, when, why* and *how* about everything.

## Laying the Groundwork for Effective Negotiation

*Under normal conditions, most people tend to see what they want to see, hear what they want to hear, and do what they want to do; in conflicts their positions become even more rigid and fixed.*

—Marc Robert



Negotiation is an ongoing process in healthcare, one you will be continually pursuing. You will be questioning your patient's healthcare providers, possibly challenging the status quo, supplying relevant information, pushing for new priorities, looking for better solutions. So let's look at the concept of negotiation and make sure we're approaching it positively.

According to the historical American business model, negotiation is an adversarial process. The conventional wisdom casts it as a three-step process: (1) Make a big impression with lots of noise, posturing, positioning, fire and brimstone. (2) Discuss actual issues of concern. (3) Bargain and compromise.

But for us as patient advocates, the reality is quite different. First, our work has no clear beginning, middle, and end, so we cannot view it as a 1-2-3 process. As long as the patient needs our help, we will continue to watch, listen, and negotiate. Moreover, if we try to make a big impression, opening with oratory, we may lose our opportunity for advocacy, possibly forever. Yelling in a hospital setting is like yelling in a library—the person who yells is shown the door! If we take an adversarial role, it suggests we are holding on to just one desired outcome: mine!

We are, in fact, discussing actual issues of concern. But, while we want a partnership, we must accept that we are not on equal footing with our patient's healthcare providers. The sooner we accept that advocates (and patients!) are viewed in a subordinate role by the healthcare establishment, the sooner we can begin to use that position in a respectful manner to invite healthcare workers to problem-solve *with* us on behalf of our patient.

But because the adversarial negotiating style is so ingrained in our business culture, it is important to consider some of its tactics and observe why they won't serve us in a patient-advocacy position.

*1. Business tactic: Negotiate on your turf, not theirs. It makes you more powerful.*

Patient advocate reality: Since our negotiations almost universally occur on the healthcare provider's turf, this is simply impossible.



*2. Business tactic: Watch for the right time. Timing works to your benefit when the other party is under deadline.*

Patient advocate reality: What are we timing? Health and healing do not function by the clock. We cannot know the outcome or timing of any intervention. (In the words of one country song, "If you want to hear God laugh, just tell Him your plans!") I found that trying to negotiate with healthcare workers when they are operating under a real or perceived timetable is a bad idea. They may, however, feel they have little time to listen to you, so be well prepared with your questions and concerns. You will earn their respect and a greater willingness to listen in the future.

*3. Business tactic: Use the clock to your advantage by squeezing the really big issues into the tightest time frame so the other party has to give up more to reach an agreement.*

Patient advocate reality: Introduce your most important issues upfront and early to allow for discussion. Whether in a doctor's office or in a hospital room, the provider has probably allocated a given number of minutes for you. If you wait until you see signals of a provider's impending departure to bring up your issue, it may be ignored. Nurses, too, often have an eye on the clock. Moreover, they are often shorthanded, and continuity can be a problem. (The very worst time to open a new subject is just before a shift change at the nursing station: departing nurses are anxious to "pass the baton" and complete the charting so they can go home; incoming nurses are anxious to learn about the preceding shift.)

***4. Business tactic: State your opening position high so when you compromise in Step 3, you stand a chance of achieving what you want.***

Patient advocate reality: While this may be true, the more practical advice is "Pick your battles." You absolutely will not gain everything you want on behalf of your patient, especially when speaking from a subordinate position with people who don't believe they need to negotiate with you! In the words of William Wordsworth, "Wisdom is oftentimes nearer when we stoop than when we soar." In today's healthcare environment, it pays to stoop. Any attempt to soar over the heads of the providers will result in a loss to your patient. The authors of *Putting Patients First* observed: "When hospital staff members are asked to list the attributes of the 'perfect patient and family,' their response is usually a passive patient with no family."[3]



***5. Business tactic: Get help/training from a contract or union negotiator with experience in adversarial situations.***

Patient advocate reality: The last thing we need is a push in the adversarial direction. Instead, we need to go beyond the concept of two opposing parties; of win versus lose, of ignoring the other's goals. One negotiation expert suggests we ask ourselves these questions: (a) How important is it to satisfy our needs? and (b) How important is it to satisfy the other person's needs?[4] When acting as an advocate, our job is to satisfy our patient's needs, keeping our own personal feelings and thoughts in check. But we must also consider our healthcare provider's need to work within a system. We can challenge that system when we must, but wherever possible, do respect the existing rules.

3 Susan Frampton, Laura Gilpin, and Patrick Charmel, "Putting Patients First," quoted by Peter Block at www.tompeters.com/slides/uploaded/Planetree_short_091706.ppt.

4 E. Wertheim, "Negotiations and Resolving Conflicts: An Overview," Northeastern University College of Business Administration, http://web.cba.neu.edu/~ewertheim/interper/negot3.htm.

***6. Business tactic: Don't tell them that you actually want to work with them, as the opposition then has no motivation to "deal" with you.***

Patient advocate reality: This advice is downright dangerous. It is vital that we show respect to our patient's providers, telling them we want to work with them on behalf of our patient. When is the last time you had a choice about which doctor or nurse tended to your patient in the hospital? The reality is that they are usually assigned. And while we can try to "drive" a doctor or nurse off our case, if we do this, we gain a reputation that makes it even harder to negotiate in the future.

***7. Business tactic: List all the issues up for discussion in a "parking lot." That way you get to see the other party's hand before the real compromises begin.***

Patient advocate reality: This us-or-them tactic has no place in patient advocacy. In business negotiations, the parties sometimes "park" related or intractable topics on a list to be revisited later. But here, "parking" a difficult issue could lead to the death of our patient. We must find a way to bring this issue out into the open in a manner that does not challenge the authority of the healthcare provider. The concept of concessions doesn't apply in patient advovacy—especially since we are discussing issues with people who are not used to negotiating with advocates and therefore don't believe we bring anything to the table.

***8. Business tactic: It takes two to negotiate. Never give up something without getting something in return.***

Patient advocate reality: The first part of this statement is absolutely true, but the second part misses the mark. If we truly do our job, we will change the minds of the healthcare providers, proving ourselves an asset to patient treatment. We must model the behavior we want from the providers, showing them how to deal with us and holding ourselves to a personal standard even higher than what we expect from others. Only in this way will we be "allowed" into the sacred halls of healthcare. Only in this way can we have any impact on behalf of our patient. In the words of Daniel Quinn, author of *Ishmael,* "Changing people's minds is something each one of us can do, wherever we are, whoever we are, whatever kind of work we're doing. Changing minds may not seem like a very dramatic or exciting challenge, but it's the challenge that the human future depends on. It's the challenge your future [and that of your patient] depends on."[5]

### *9. Business tactic: Once you have a deal, take advantage of the agreement and ask for "a little more."*

Patient advocate reality: Introducing a new issue right after securing an agreement with a healthcare worker will likely be perceived as greedy or even as a betrayal, particularly if that person went to bat for you. It will, in any case, make that person less willing to negotiate with you again. So stay focused on the big things. The little things may take care of themselves, or perhaps you can address them personally.



Here's an example. While Bill was comatose and breathing with a ventilator, we faced almost hourly crises, sometimes with as many as ten healthcare workers needed at his side. During the rare quiet moments, I noticed that his lips were becoming chapped, almost to the point of bleeding. This was obviously not life-threatening, but if and when Bill awoke, it would be painful. When I asked the nurse about it, she told me the only lip emollient on hand was alcohol-based: a combustion risk near the ventilator. Were non-alcohol-based lip treatments available? I asked, and she said yes, through health stores. After thinking a moment, I decided not to ask the nurse for any special favors. I was way more concerned about her life-saving skills. Although I was terrified to leave Bill's side, I made a trip to a local health store for the emollient, adding this to the list of things I could do personally for my patient.

Ask yourself how each person views you. Your primary care physician, who expects to maintain a long-term relationship with you, may take a more cooperative position than, for example, a hospital doctor, consulting physician, or nurse, whose contact with you will be minimal. As an advocate, you must try to set the stage for "win/win" relationship-building negotiations.

---

5 Daniel Quinn, "The New Renaissance," address delivered to the University of Texas Health Science Center, Houston, Mar. 7, 2002, http://www.mnforsustain.org/quinn_d_new_renaissance.htm.

Your job is to facilitate consensus so that everyone—but especially your patient—wins. You are there to follow the healthcare system's rules but not to play their game. You must know:

- what your patient wants and is willing to accept
- what you want and are willing to accept without compromising your ethics
- what each healthcare worker wants and is willing to accept



If this sounds like hard work, that's because it is! Especially difficult is the act of setting aside your personal wishes if they differ from the patient's. I wanted my husband to survive. But today I wonder: if Bill had known what lay ahead, would he have shared my life-saving goal for him? Some patient advocates have to deal with this very issue.

In any case, stay creative and open in negotiations, keeping these in mind:

- Your approach: Be willing to "switch gears" midstream when new information is provided.
- Your research: Continuously research your patient's condition and related topics. No doctor can keep up with all the changes occurring daily in medicine, and the medical staff doesn't have time to educate you. It is your job to stay informed and share your knowledge as appropriate.
- Your behavior: Because you are probably viewed as the subordinate in the negotiation, find the power in that position and bring it to bear.
- Your solutions: Asking healthcare workers how they would solve a problem is a great start. You will learn something about the treatment as well as the individual, which may make it easier to resolve the difference.
- Your listening: If you cannot listen—both to what is said and not said—help your patient find another advocate. If your feelings are plugging up your ears, you can no longer function effectively. You must be aware enough of yourself and your triggers to recognize this and take the needed steps.

Mary Parker Follett reminds us that "Coercive power is the curse of the universe; coactive power, the enrichment and advancement of every human soul."

Negotiations occur when there are problems to be solved. Nature seems to have had this process in place even before humankind's appearance. Nature uses all materials, adapts to climate and environmental changes, and flows with the seasons. "Nature, imaginative by necessity, has already solved many of the problems with which we are grappling," says Janine Benyus in her book *Biomimicry.*[6] Her "nine basic laws of the circle of life," shown in italics below, are amended here with my thoughts on patient advocacy.[7]



1. *Nature runs on sunlight.* Know what fuels you and what drains you. Take a walk outside when you get stuck in a negotiation or other issue.
2. *Nature uses only the energy it needs.* Go to the mat only when needed. Constant negotiations drain everybody.
3. *Nature fits form to function.* Make noise only for the big issues. Otherwise, speak calmly but with passion. Often the whisperer has the loudest voice.
4. *Nature recycles everything.* Acknowledge a provider who gives you what has been requested. We don't get repetitive behavior without rewards.
5. *Nature rewards cooperation.* Remind yourself that we are all in this to help the patient.
6. *Nature banks on diversity.* The healthcare staff are the treatment experts, but the patient is the local expert on his or her own body and wishes. All views must be valued and heard, even unconventional ones.
7. *Nature curbs excesses from within.* Seek a balanced treatment plan—balanced in favor of serving the patient's wishes. Make sure healthcare staff are aware of any living will or "do not resuscitate" orders, lest the drive to save a life overwhelm the patient's desires.
8. *Nature taps the power of limits.* You are attempting to negotiate where others have feared to tread. Organizations and individuals resist change, and what we do is all about change. We are seeking a voice within a system that

6 Janine M. Benyus, *Biomimicry: Innovation Inspired by Nature* (New York: HarperCollins, 1997).

7 Ibid. Used with permission.

protects itself at all costs, a system that believes that: (a) Advocates are incapable of understanding, (b) Our role should be one of passivity, (c) The patient has rights (although the system rarely delivers on this belief), and (d) Death is a failure, even if that is the desire of the patient. If this is not tapping the power of limits, I don't know what is.

We would do well to travel in Nature's footsteps.



## Negotiating Change: Five Personal Steps

*If you want to make enemies, try to change something.*

—Woodrow Wilson

*Life is either a daring adventure, or nothing. To keep our faces toward change and behave like free spirits in the presence of fate is strength undefeatable.*

—Helen Keller, *Let Us Have Faith*

Hospitals are first and foremost systems. A system is an entity that consists of both content (tasks, policies, rules, jobs) and processes (tradition, practice, unwritten norms, expectations, ways of doing things). As an entity it is complete in itself. A system is made up of parts, and the system is larger than the sum of its parts. A system is separate from the people who populate it: it existed before those people, and it will continue after they are gone. Think of corporations, universities, workplaces, governments—and hospitals.

Systems contain within themselves entire worldviews. Imagine looking into a snow globe—there is a world within the glass. Systems are expected to make sense of everything that happens within them. And the way a system uses new information depends on how open or closed it is. In closed systems, information that does not validate the current system will often be disregarded. In other words, closed systems tend to maintain the status quo.

As patient advocates, we are often questioning the status quo. When we ask for something for our patient, when we ask a care provider to consider a different approach, when we bring something new to that person's attention—we are asking that care provider to consider making a change. And change is often tough for human beings.

Most of us are familiar with the "five stages of grief" originally presented by Elisabeth Kübler-Ross, MD, in her book *On Death and Dying*. But these stages have far broader applications: they can even be considered the "five stages of change." It is now understood that anyone undergoing any major change can expect to go through the five-step cycle in some way.



### *Stages in Adapting to Change*

Kübler-Ross identified these five stages, and we can apply them to any kind of change, including the process of illness and healing:

- denial
- anger
- bargaining
- depression
- acceptance[8]

Not only will your patient experience these stages, so will the patient's family, friends, caregivers, and healthcare workers—and so will you, as you process your feelings about your patient and the outcomes of your advocacy.

My personal experience has shown that this sequence can be different for men and women.

Men tend to cycle like this:

- denial
- anger, anger, anger: for men, this feeling is socially acceptable—they may hide other feelings behind it and can get stuck here
- bargaining: typically silent and inside oneself
- depression: for men, this is less socially acceptable, so they may ignore it, rush through it, or mask it as anger
- acceptance

8 Elisabeth Kübler-Ross, *On Death and Dying* (New York: Touchstone, 1969).

Women tend to cycle like this:

- denial
- depression, depression, depression: for women, this feeling is socially acceptable, so they can get stuck here
- bargaining: this can help motivate women out of depression or can serve as a landmark that they have moved through it
- anger: for women, this is less socially acceptable, so they may ignore it, rush through it, or mask it
- acceptance



Let's look at a few more things we know about how people handle these stages.

- This is not a straight-line process. All of you will weave in and out of each of these stages many times: patient, family and friends, caregivers, healthcare workers, and you.
- You can and will be "hauled backwards" by certain events or trigger phrases. But each time you revert to an earlier stage, you will process it faster and move on more quickly.
- People who are inward-focused may suffer from what I call the "beachball effect." They hold their changing feelings inside, like puffs of air in a beachball. What eventually happens? It blows up, often with no warning. (Think of how often a person who "went postal" is described as "quiet and withdrawn.")
- The people around us—spouse, family, friends—may be in varying stages. For example, I may be fine with what is happening and my spouse may be angry. Or I may be depressed and my spouse is telling me to "get over it." Get the picture?
- Acting "as if" helps all of us move on. Try going through the motions of the next stage, and you might just find yourself there for real.

William Bridges, author of *Managing Transitions,* has a theory about change: he defines the stages as "ending, exploration, new beginnings." Or, said another way: frozen, unfrozen, refrozen. However you choose to view this model, there is chaos in the middle of it—a chaos that Bridges also calls the "wilderness."[9] You may feel out of control, anxious, depressed, lost. This is normal! Seek help if you get stuck. Do you have access to a counselor or an Employee Assistance Program? Use them if you need them; they can be invaluable.



But we can also cope with this chaos, this wilderness, by analyzing and using our "spheres of influence."[10] This gives us tools not only for now, but for a lifetime.

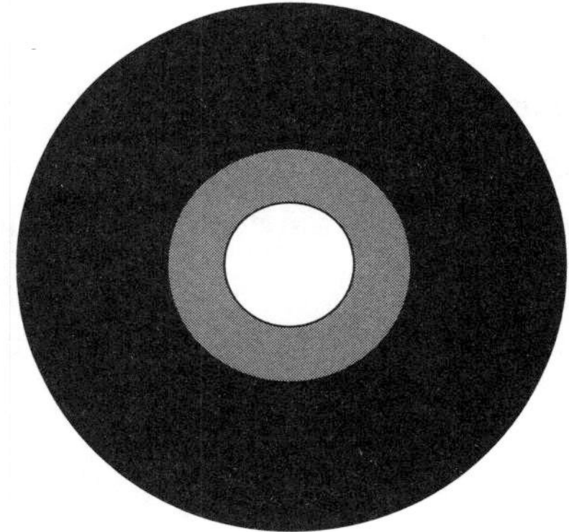

***WHITE** =* ***I can control***
***GRAY** =* ***I can influence***
***BLACK** =* ***I cannot control or influence***

First, look at the white circle. What do you have total control over? Yourself: your own feelings and behavior. We can always control how we react to events. For patients and patient advocates, sometimes this is the only thing we

9 William Bridges, *Managing Transitions: Making the Most Out of Change* (New York: Perseus Books, 1991).

10 Graphic adapted from David L. Hultgran, "Spheres of Influence: Doing What You Can Do," *Training and Development Journal*, July 1989.

can manage. We can be miserable, confused, angry, blaming others—or we can take control of ourselves and decide how we want to be.

Now let's look to the gray circle: our sphere of influence. In some areas of our lives we may not have total control, but we have influence—perhaps with particular people: family, co-workers, community groups, maybe even our patient. And we may have more influence than we think. We may also find that as we take more responsibility within our white circle, our gray circle begins to expand. As we do good work, keep a good attitude, and prove our abilities, our influence grows: that is a key for advocates.



What about the black circle? In this sphere we have neither control nor influence. Some things are given: for example, hospital policy, the rules of the insurance system, the course of our patient's disease—these are beyond our scope. Experience teaches us that if we focus energy on fighting these "givens," our actual sphere of influence—the gray area—shrinks.

Remember, advocacy is 90 percent attitude. If people are "taking your temperature," you are probably "leaking," trying to operate outside your personal sphere of influence. Step back. This is not the time to pursue a negotiation!

Try this mantra.

*I am responsible for the input. I am not responsible for the outcome.*

If you do what you can do when you can, the rest is out of your hands, including the life of your patient.

Angeles Arrien, in her work with various cultures and eras, has explored the accumulated wisdom of indigenous tribal methods for dealing with and solving conflict. She summarizes these methods as four principles, calling it "The Four-Fold Way" in her book of the same title.

1. Show up, or choose to be present.
2. Pay attention to what has heart and meaning.
3. Tell the truth without blame or judgment.
4. Be open to outcome, not attached to outcome.[11]

11 Angeles Arrien, *The Four-Fold Way.*

What do these mean for us as advocates?

***1. Show up, or choose to be present.***

We must be fully in the now—physically, mentally, emotionally, and spiritually. We own our feelings and acknowledge them, at least to ourselves. We do not act from them, as strong feelings can hamper our communication with others. But we can selectively share them: I found that when I told healthcare providers how I was feeling, barriers melted in many cases. Ignoring our feelings invites disaster, for our interactions as well as for our personal health.



***2. Pay attention to what has heart and meaning.***

Earlier we noted the wisdom of picking your battles as a patient advocate. Of equal importance is representing what has heart and meaning *for your patient.* Acknowledge internally what has heart and meaning for you, but do not base your communications on it. You are there to represent another, not yourself. For your own integrity, you must remain consistent in this mission.

***3. Tell the truth without blame or judgment.***

Take a factual, practical approach when communicating with healthcare providers. Given their scientific training, they are more likely to respond to "just the facts, ma'am"—the newspaper reporter's dictum. When I took this approach, my comments were far better received and less likely to meet resistance. Even when mistakes have been made—both of commission and omission—avoid blaming. Once you engage in the "blame game," walls go up.

***4. Be open to outcome, not attached to outcome.***

We can only operate within our sphere of influence. What is best for the patient? What are the patient's wishes? When we act with these questions always in mind, we can rest assured that we have truly acted on the patient's behalf. The rest is in God's hands.

Clarissa Pinkola Estés gives us a picture of what advocacy looks like when implemented. While this is an assignment she gave the world, I quote it here as the assignment I give to each of you:

> I assign you to be a beautiful, good, kind, awakened, soulful person, a true work of art as we say, *ser humano*, a true human being. In a world filled with so much darkness, such a soul shines like gold; can be seen from a far distance; is dramatically different.
>
> . . . Anything you do from the soulful self will help lighten the burdens of the world. Anything. You have no idea what the smallest word, the tiniest generosity can cause to be set in motion. Be outrageous in forgiving. Be dramatic in reconciling. Mistakes? Back up and make them as right as you can, then move on. Be off the charts in kindness. In whatever you are called to, strive to be devoted to it in all aspects large and small. Fall short? Try again. Mastery is made in increments, not in leaps. Be brave, be fierce, be visionary. Mend the parts of the world that are 'within your reach.' To strive to live this way is the most dramatic gift you can ever give to the world.
>
> Consider yourselves assigned.[12]



## The Disease Called Denial: A Call to Action

> *The only people for me are the mad ones, the ones who are mad to live, mad to talk, mad to be saved, desirous of everything at the same time, the ones who never yawn or say a commonplace thing, but burn, burn, burn, burn like fabulous yellow roman candles exploding like spiders across the stars . . .*
>
> —Jack Kerouac, *Beat Generation*

Denial is one of the strongest and most destructive of human habits. And it can be systemic, too, with many people colluding either consciously or unconsciously. In the United States, systemic denial is nowhere more visible than in healthcare. Denial *of* healthcare is a different matter—that is, the refusal of treatment or insurance coverage for a patient. Here we're looking at our collective denial about the state of the whole healthcare system, and how that denial helps maintain the status quo.

12 Clarissa Pinkola Estés, "Today's Assignment: A Prescription From Dr. E.," Dr. Estés, http://www.mavenproductions.com/estes_cpe3_window.html. Reprinted with permission.

Our medical institutions, practitioners, and we as healthcare consumers all suffer from denial—the disease that postpones action because we won't even admit the problems. And if we don't face it, U.S. medical care will likely drop even lower in the World Health Organization's worldwide ranking: it was 37th in 2000.[13] As Dr. Christopher Murray, director of WHO's Global Programme on Evidence for Health Policy, noted in that year:



> The position of the United States is one of the major surprises of the new rating system. Basically, you die earlier and spend more time disabled if you're an American rather than a member of most other advanced countries.[14]

Of course, denial has its positive functions. For example, we generally live without thinking about the fact that we could die at any moment. At times denial may also offer us temporary solace while we gather strength. But ultimately denial prevents us from addressing what needs addressing. And ignoring the state of U.S. healthcare today is like ignoring the elephant in your living room.

Our entire healthcare system today is in pain. By definition, pain hurts, and we prefer not to experience it. We tend live our lives avoiding pain and seeking satisfaction and pleasure (or at least ways to escape from pain). But pain is a symptom of a problem, a warning we must heed in our own best interests. In the case of our healthcare system, the temptation is to ignore the challenge and try to go numb. We try to invalidate the evidence of the problem; we simply defend the status quo. When we do, we may temporarily feel safe, but our hurt and pain will return again and again until we face it. Ignoring the hurt and pain disempowers us. Facing the hurt and pain empowers us.

But it requires passion for truth, and it means removing our rose-colored glasses. Our belief that healthcare workers have a corner on saving lives is comforting for patients and advocates, tempting us to relinquish all our power to them. The belief of many healthcare workers that they are best qualified to heal is comforting for them, tempting them to assume all the power in their

---

13 World Health Organization, "WHO Issues New Healthy Life Expectancy Rankings," http://www.who.int/inf-pr-2000/en/pr2000-life.html.

14 Ibid.

relationship with patients and advocates. But both of these beliefs can act as blinders and prevent meaningful communication. They can also be used to defend all sorts of behaviors.



Thus our ability to change how we think about ourselves and others is a critical part of healing our healthcare system. When we fall back on the roles of "us and them," expert and nonexpert, with no need for collaboration, we do ourselves a disservice. That black-and-white world may offer us a false security, but there is no healing. Patients and their advocates must become full partners in their own healthcare.

Here are just a few examples of the effects of our denial about healthcare—practitioners, administrators, and consumers alike.

- The U.S. healthcare system can bankrupt its own citizens. High out-of-pocket costs of prescription drugs contribute to about half the nation's personal bankrupties.[15] And many insurance policies pay only up to a lifetime maximum: often a dollar amount that can, with today's technology, easily be exceeded by a patient with complex medical needs.
- About 44 million Americans have no medical insurance at all.[16]
- Multiple-doctor care is often poorly coordinated: a real problem when many specialists are involved. Relatively few university and teaching hospitals have hospitalists, doctors who specifically coordinate multiple-doctor care and keep the whole patient in mind. Absent the hospitalist, the patient needs a very good advocate.
- Hospital understaffing is partly a function of the broken system. Hospital administrators are held accountable for profits, but they have no control over the money flow into the system—that is, through insurers. All they can do is control costs, leading to understaffing and under-equipping.

---

15 David U. Himmelstein, Elizabeth Warren, Deborah Thorne, and Steffie Woolhandler, "MarketWatch: Illness and Injury as Contributors to Bankruptcy," *Health Affairs*, Feb. 2, 2005, http://content.healthaffairs.org/cgi/content/full/hlthaff.w5.63/DC1.

16 John D. Dingell, "Subcommittee on Oversight and Investigations Hearing on 'A Review of Hospital Billing and Collection Practices,'" Committee on Energy and Commerce, June 24, 2004, http://energycommerce.house.gov/press/108st122.shtml.

- Hospital staff "patient advocates" may have a conflict of interest. They are employed by the hospital administration, but are supposed to represent the patient's interests.
- Doctors themselves may have a conflict of interest. HMOs often pay doctors financial incentives for limiting their referrals—referrals that can greatly improve patient care.
- Patients are underinformed. Healthcare workers are chronically rushed, with no time to ensure that patients understand their treatment—a right granted them in the Patient Rights Statement.
- Medical terminology sometimes obscures the truth. When providers refer to a "nosocomial" or "iatrogenic" infection, they mean it was hospital-acquired or caused by a doctor's care. But using these terms with laypeople helps them hide their own role in the transmission of infections.
- Hospital errors do occur—frequently—but are rarely apologized for, despite many surveys showing patients are far less likely to sue if they are informed in a humane and responsible manner.



As long as we stay in denial, these problems will continue. When will we wake up? When the call to truth overpowers self-deception. When the call for healing overpowers the calls to conform. I am calling for truth in healthcare. I am calling for healing in healthcare. And I am calling for all of us to step forward with our truth and work collectively to heal this healthcare system.

Angeles Arrien tells us that there are three universal processes in working through change: work with the self, work with another, and collective work.[17] The first process determines our readiness. We must answer the question, "Is my self-worth as strong as my self-critic?" Only when the answer is yes can we proceed to work through this change. The second process involves one-on-one work, which teaches us about intimacy. (And what is more intimate than sharing the care of our body with another person?) The third process leads us to collective

17 The source for all these passages is Angeles Arrien, *Change, Conflict, and Resolution from a Cross-Cultural Perspective.*

work, which teaches us about family, community, and unfinished business. And again, healthcare intervention almost always includes those elements.

Dr. Arrien also tells us that the majority of the world's problem-solving is done through collective work, and that is the call of the twenty-first century. This is not the work of any individual or small organization. The U.S. healthcare problem can only be solved by the collective, and we all have a role to play in that solution.



How? We can find lessons in these observations of migrating geese, lessons that illustrate the benefits of the collective. As referred to by Dr. Arrien, these observations follow, together with my comments.

*Geese get where they are going in formation 71% faster than if they went individually.* ***Lesson***—*If you are going somewhere, you will get there faster if you join a group of people that are going in the same direction. If you are going in a group, it helps immensely to all go in the same direction!*

We all need to move toward a system dedicated to the best interests of the patient, according to the patient! Practitioners may think they know those interests—but have they ever asked patients what they want? We need a system where providers spend time with each patient, ask about wants and needs, ask how care could be improved, encourage living wills or advance directives, and listen. "Open-ended listening; nondefensive, neutral, and empathic responses; silence; and frequent regular interaction with family and patient from a designated physician can encourage trust and help lead to a diminution or resolution of denial," in the words of Paul Rousseau, MD.[18] We want a system where patients are encouraged to stay healthy, to complete a living will or advance directive—no matter what their age—and to collaborate in their own care.

18 Paul Rousseau, "Death Denial," *Journal of Clinical Oncology* 18, no. 23 (December 2000), http://jco.ascopubs.org/cgi/content/full/18/23/3998.

*If a goose drops out of a formation, he will try as hard as he can to rejoin the formation.* ***Lesson****—If you are as smart as a goose, you will try as hard as you can to stick with those going in your direction and you will notice how very hard it is to go alone.*

The people in our lives—family, friends, and others—are our "formation" of mutual support. Going to the hospital as a patient is a scary proposition. If you know anyone who is being admitted to a hospital, offer to help. There are so many things patients and their advocates need that even if you cannot be present frequently, you can still make a contribution. Since often we cannot directly pay back the people who provide us with favors and strength, we can return the favor to others in need. What goes around, comes around.



*When the lead goose gets tired, he drops out of the lead and rejoins the group further back in the formation. Another goose always moves up to take the lead.* ***Lesson****—It is better to share the most difficult tasks than to depend on one person all the time. Good leaders recognize that they can't do the leadership role all the time and that they need to rotate that position.*

Patient advocates must share their responsibility: no single person can or should serve at the bedside 24/7. To try to do so is to act from denial. Acting on behalf of another and heeding their wishes carries great responsibility and stress. All caregivers must also care for themselves. And ideally, discussions and planning for these roles should be done in the calm state of good health.

*When one of the geese drops out of the formation due to injury or illness, two other geese will drop out of the formation and stay with him until he has either recovered or died. They will then try to catch up with the original formation or join another formation.* ***Lesson****—Always provide help to those that are in trouble. Stick with them until the problem is resolved. Don't break up the whole formation because of the obstacle.*

Learn both to offer support and to accept it. Let others help you when you need it. And, as a patient advocate, stand by your patient. Defend your patient's preferences even if you disagree with them—end-of-life issues included.

*Geese in the back of the formation honk to encourage the ones up front to do their very best.* ***Lesson***—*Things go much better if you give words of encouragement to those who lead.*

We will not change our healthcare system by tearing down its practitioners. It is staffed by loving and caring individuals who have been trained to save lives. To change does not necessarily mean to change everything. It often means making constant, incremental changes over time. The result we want is a healthcare system dedicated to serving the patient first. Meanwhile, we can support the positive things that happen in our healthcare system every day. And, as we discover answers or clues for positive change, we can step forward, speak our truth, and offer to help.

# LESSONS IN CAREGIVING

*There are only four kinds of people in the world: those who have been caregivers; those who are currently caregivers; those who will be caregivers; those who will need caregivers.*

—Rosalynn Carter

I was a failure at giving care. I did not fail my husband, I failed myself. I failed to care for myself while giving care to my husband. And this is a common failure among caregivers, as I realized when I began to read about others' experiences. Misery does love company, but I almost died learning this lesson.

When I say the word "failure," to what am I referring? According to long-term care-planning expert Thomas Day, a typical progression for long-term caregivers may unfold as follows:

- 1 to 18 months: Things are fine, I am fine, and help is available.
- 20 to 36 months: I'm not fine and need meds to function, I'm alone, I can't cope, and little help is available.

- 38 to 50 months: I'm not well, there are too many decisions for me to make, and if something doesn't change, *I* will need a caregiver soon.[1]

During Bill's illness and his years of recovery, I became a candidate for long-term care myself, and only avoided it by finally "abandoning my post." That's how it felt, in my guilt-ridden view at the time. But many of us thrown into caregiving do not know where our boundaries are, and we try to do things beyond our ability. In my case, I had the expertise but lacked the stamina—understandably!—to sustain my care for Bill over six years of recovery time. But at the time, I felt I had failed. Today, my perspective is different because I now recognize that what made me good at advocacy doomed my caregiving.



As an advocate, I worked on behalf of my patient to get *others* to provide a service or take action. As a caregiver, *I* additionally had to provide the service or take the action myself. Each activity, advocacy and caregiving, is a full-time job. How can one person be expected to do both, especially over the long haul? But then, who is ever trained to be what I became? An informal caregiver, according to one definition, is a "family member, friend, neighbor or church member who provides unpaid care out of love, respect, obligation or friendship to a disabled person."[2] Without these people, many patients and disabled individuals in this country would either lack care or overburden the medical community.

## The State of Giving Care in the United States

How many informal caregivers are there in the United States? According to the National Alliance for Caregiving/MetLife, "depending on the definition of caregiving, estimates range from 20 million to 50 million people. This represents about 20% of the total population providing part- or full-time care."[3]

1 Thomas Day, "About Caregiving," Long Term Care Link, http://www.longtermcarelink.net/eldercare/caregiving.htm (passage adapted from Washington State Aging and Disabilities Services Administration text). Day is director of the National Care Planning Council.

2 Ibid.

3 Metropolitan Life Insurance Company, "MetLife Study of Employer Costs for Working Caregivers," 1997, http://www.metlife.com/WPSAssets/14002396171048285176V1FEmployer%20Costs%20study%20.pdf.

In 2005, *HealthDay News* reported that adults who care for a sick or disabled family member "often have medical problems of their own, lack health insurance and are stressed by medical bills. 45 percent of the caregivers have one or more chronic health problems, compared to 24 percent of those who are not caregivers. It looks like they are having a difficult time."[4]



I would say so! Various surveys over the last few years reveal the following trends in caregiving:

- About two-thirds of caregivers are women.
- Most caregivers are between the ages of 50 and 64.
- Compared to non-caregivers, about 15 percent more caregivers have difficulty finding medical insurance because of their own medical problems.
- The average amount of time an individual provides care for another is four years.
- For about 10 percent of caregivers, the responsibility means they are unable to hold down a fulltime job.
- Informal caregivers lose about $660,000 in wage wealth over their lifetime because of work sacrifices.[5]

What can we do differently for our own well-being, and ultimately for our loved one's well-being? Caregivers must make sure their own needs are known and taken care of. Let's consider some of these ways.

- **Explore work alternatives.** If you have a job, talk with your employer. Perhaps your work schedule can be made flexible to accommodate appointments and your own "shifts" as caregiver. Perhaps you can work from home.

4 Kathleen Doheny, "Caregivers Face Major Medical Hurdles of Their Own," *HealthDay News*, Aug. 24, 2005, http://www.healthywomen.org/resources/womenshealthinthenews/dbhealthnews/caregiversfacemajormedicalhurdlesoftheirown.

5 Points 1–3: Kathleen Doheny, "Caregivers Face Major Medical Hurdles of Their Own"; points 4–5: Metropolitan Life Insurance Company, "MetLife Study of Employer Costs for Working Caregivers"; point 6: Family Caregiver Alliance, "2007 Policy Statement," 2007, http://www.caregiver.org/caregiver/jsp/content_node.jsp?nodeid=883.

(The advantage at home is that you're still available to provide care. The disadvantage at home is that you're still available to provide care—and going to a job can give you a needed break.) Perhaps you can share your job with someone else. Many companies have begun to recognize the issue by offering unpaid FMLA leave, as provided for by the Family and Medical Leave Act, for sustained time off for senior care and for unexpected needs as well as for baby care. Resources are also available through nonprofit and for-profit organizations.

- **Ask for help.** Families should share in caregiving, and a family conference can help organize tasks, schedules, and ways to include older children. Perhaps neighbors can help with transportation and shopping. As a caregiver for her husband, my mother kept an ongoing list of tasks that needed doing; whenever someone offered to help, she went to the list.
- **Plan early for caregiving help,** *before* your loved one comes home from the hospital—even if a quick recovery is expected. Medical needs often do not end with discharge from the hospital. Plan for plenty of help: you are worth it!
- **Do something just for you every day** even if it is just a short break.
- **Exercise** for at least thirty minutes, three times a week. It helps discharge stress and releases endorphins—those natural "feel good" chemicals.
- **Eat healthy:** "eat closer to the earth," as my dietician friend Karen tells me—meals made from whole ingredients. I look for fairly low-carb, low-calorie foods with lots of protein and without hydrogenated fats, sugar, salts, or chemical preservatives or additives. (I don't like to cook, so I ate poorly during Bill's illness. Things got better when he started cooking again.)
- **Subscribe** to caregiving newsletters or listservs for advice and support. These are some of the best ones I have discovered.
  - ✓ www.caregiver.com
  - ✓ www.caregiver.org (nonprofit)
  - ✓ www.thefamilycaregiver.org

✓ www.caps4caregivers.org

✓ www.48friend.org

✓ www.wellspouse.org

✓ www.familycaregiving101.org

- **Join a support group for caregivers.** The local healthcare community, the Area Agency on Aging, and even your doctor may be able to make recommendations.



- **Get professional help if you need it**—and even if you don't (because you really do). For me, it helped me process feelings such as guilt, despair, anger, frustration, and many more. And processing those feelings with Bill himself would not have been good for our relationship.

- **Practice "Caregiver Self-Advocacy,"** as recommended by the National Family Caregivers Association and the National Alliance for Caregiving. The four principles listed below will help you set boundaries and care for yourself. (For more information visit www.familycaregiving101.org.)

  1. Choose to take charge of your life.
  2. Love, honor and value yourself.
  3. Seek, accept, and at times demand help.
  4. Stand up and be counted.[6]

Caregiving can be very fulfilling if you keep these points in mind.

Family caregiving is a critical piece of our long-term care system. In fact, "family and other unpaid caregivers provide nearly 80 percent of all long-term care in this country. We also know that the less income a caregiver has, the more stress he or she is likely to experience *and* that caregivers use prescription drugs for depression, anxiety and insomnia two to three times as often as the rest of

6 National Family Caregivers Association (NFCA) and National Alliance for Caregiving (NAC) "Four Messages to Live By," Family Caregiving 101, http://www.familycaregiving101.org/manage/messages.cfm#3.

the population."[7] With the influx of baby boomers into the senior category, it is anticipated that by 2050, there will be one person requiring care for every four caregivers, a far cry from the 1:11 ratio we saw in 1990.[8] We need to wake up as a society and address the needs of caregivers today!

Here are some resources for caregiving; see also the Resources section.



- National Family Caregivers Association (NFCA) website at www.thefamilycaregiver.org
- National Care Planning Council website, *Long Term Care Link,* at www.longtermcarelink.net
- Health and Age website, www.healthandage.com; (see *Caregivers' Center)*
- HealthDay News at www.healthday.com
- Aging and Disability Services Administration at www.aasa.dshs.wa.gov

---

7 Orange County Office on Aging, "Condition of Older Adults: 2003 Report," 2003, http://www.officeonaging.ocgov.com/PDFs/Conditions%20Report%20Section%202.pdf.

8 Dean Gallagher, "Caring for Our Caregivers," *Elder Update* 10, no. 6 (Sept. 2000), Florida Department of Elder Affairs, http://elderaffairs.state.fl.us/english/EUoldissues/doeaeu0009.pdf.

## The Fearless Caregiver Manifesto: How to Get the Best Care for Your Loved One and Still Have a Life of Your Own

Reprinted with permission from Gary Barg, author of *The Fearless Caregiver: How to Get the Best Care for Your Loved One and Still Have a Life of Your Own* and editor-in-chief and publisher of *caregiver.com.*

I will fearlessly assess my personal strengths and weaknesses, work diligently to bolster my weaknesses and to graciously recognize my strengths.



I will fearlessly make my voice be heard with regard to my loved one's care and be a strong ally to those professional caregivers committed to caring for my loved one and a fearless shield against those not committed to caring for my loved one.

I will fearlessly not sign or approve anything I do not understand, and will steadfastly request the information I need until I am satisfied with the explanations.

I will fearlessly ensure that all of the necessary documents are in place in order for my wishes and my loved one's wishes to be met in case of a medical emergency. These will include *Durable Medical Powers of Attorney, Wills, Trusts* and *Living Wills.*

I will fearlessly learn all I can about my loved one's healthcare needs and become an integral member of his or her medical care team.

I will fearlessly seek out other caregivers or care organizations and join an appropriate support group; I realize that there is strength in numbers and will not isolate myself from those who are also caring for their loved ones.

I will fearlessly care for my physical and emotional health as well as I care for my loved one's, I will recognize the signs of my own exhaustion and depression, and I will allow myself to take respite breaks and to care for myself on a regular basis.

I will fearlessly develop a personal support system of friends and family and remember that others also love my loved one and are willing to help if I let them know what they can do to support my caregiving.

I will fearlessly honor my loved one's wishes, as I know them to be, unless these wishes endanger their health or mine.

I will fearlessly acknowledge when providing appropriate care for my loved one becomes impossible either because of his or her condition or my own, and seek other solutions for my loved one's caregiving needs.

# LESSONS IN MONEY MATTERS

For patients in the U.S. healthcare system, financial matters can get complicated very quickly. The amounts of money and the volume of paperwork can both be daunting. But for advocates, many of the abilities that serve you at the bedside will serve you here as well: problem-solving skills, vigilant attention to detail, and willingness both to seek help and to question authority. Let's look first at some general strategies for handling the unexpected expenses, then at some tips for understanding hospital bills.

## Strategies for Handling Unexpected Medical Expenses

Anyone who pays for health insurance or has stayed even briefly in a hospital can attest to the frightening rise in the cost of healthcare. Bill's medical expenses almost bankrupted us, even with "full" medical coverage. They continued to haunt him for six years: his credit record was flawed by nonpayment of a $200 hospital invoice. Bill is still recovering, and his out-of-pocket medical bills now average $20,000 a year: the cost of his illness's damage to his body. My own yearly health expenses are not far behind: the cost of Bill's illness to *my* body.

What can we do when unexpected medical expenses arise? Here are some ideas. Most of these I tried myself; some I have more recently discovered and believe they could be helpful.

**Use the expertise of family and friends.** My brother-in-law is an accountant and I enlisted his help in matching up medical bills with the Explanation of Benefits forms (also known as EOBs) from the insurance company. He tracked discrepancies and suggested strategies for delaying payments without incurring the wrath of the providers. Later, Bill's employer helped strongarm an insurance carrier that had failed to deliver (after that employer had ended their partnership).

**Apply for Social Security benefits where possible.** I applied the very second Bill was eligible, and the fact that he was on full life support and diagnosed with end-stage kidney disease speeded up the actual payments. (That, plus the fact that I burst into tears in the clerk's office and she took pity on me.) Many Social Security claims are denied, however. If you believe your patient is eligible but is denied, consider talking with an attorney who specializes in this type of law. With an attorney's help, my brother-in-law received the benefits he was initially denied. This process took some time, however, so don't rely on this income for immediate needs.

**To resolve insurance claims, talk with management and take notes.** When I began to insist on itemized insurance bills, at first I spent hours on the phone with multiple first-line clerks who could not grasp the complexity of Bill's situation. Then, rather than consume more medication myself, I began to request to speak to a supervisor, ratcheting it up to a demand if necessary. I was finally connected with a truly effective, wonderful woman who then worked hand in hand with me for over a year to resolve outstanding bills. She joined me on the phone with five collection agencies, verifying that neither the insurance carrier nor Bill and Jari Buck would pay any claims without itemized proof of every expense. Ultimately, four sets of claims were withdrawn and a fifth was resolved in our favor. Another tip: take notes when on the phone. Record the date and time, person, and outcome of the conversation. It will help you reconstruct your case if you need to—with a collection agency, for example.

**Consider disability for yourself if you are an overextended caregiver.** I applied for these benefits myself during Bill's illness: I was having such trouble coping emotionally that I could not work and was on medication. Initially my claim was rejected, but I appealed, and when the company learned my story (from my primary care physician), I was approved and drew benefits for eight months. That revenue didn't match what I could have earned, but it helped.

**For a patient receiving disability, check with lenders for help with payments.** Some loan or credit card policies may waive certain home-loan or charge card payments during the period of disability. If you have such a policy, contact the company, request information, and file a claim.



**Look into assistance from the Patient Advocate Foundation.** This national nonprofit organization "serves as an active liaison between the patient and their insurer, employer and/or creditors to resolve insurance, job retention and/or debt crisis matters relative to their diagnosis through case managers, doctors and attorneys."[1] Patients with any of the diagnoses shown here may qualify; help may also be available in the case of secondary issues resulting from cancer treatment. Visit www.patientadvocate.org or call 800-532-5274.

- autoimmune disorders
- breast cancer
- colon cancer
- diabetes
- kidney cancer
- lung cancer
- lymphoma
- macular degeneration
- malignant brain tumors
- pancreatic cancer
- prostate cancer
- sarcoma

1 Patient Advocate Foundation, "Patient Advocate Foundation Mission Statement," http://www.patientadvocate.org.

**Negotiate payment plans with your health-related creditors.** Most will do this only for large amounts. But some may let you pay off even a small debt over time with no interest, provided you do not miss a monthly payment. Others may refer you to a business partner who will set up a plan and charge interest. Either way can save you from up-front payment in full.



**Ask for lower minimum payments on your credit cards.** It is worth trying; contact your credit card companies and see if they will work with you. I have had mixed luck with this, but I am now a customer for life with the companies that cut me some slack; I closed many of my other accounts.

**Consider enrolling in a credit monitoring service** for at least a year after incurring any healthcare debt. For a nominal fee, the service will alert you if anything negative shows up on your credit report. You can then act to resolve it—rather than learning about it later when you are turned down for additional credit.

**Contact other professionals for ideas.** Your spiritual leader may know of no-cost or low-cost services that could help you. Hospital chaplains and hospital social workers may be particularly knowledgeable.

**Look into "disease-specific" organizations.** If your patient has a disease, go online and search for national and local organizations, for example, the American Diabetes Association or the National Cancer Institute. Although these organizations will not give you money, they often have a network of affiliates who may be able to provide free goods or services. They may also offer referrals to other medical providers and local support groups.

**Consider what you can sell.** One option is eBay, or find a person or organization who will list your goods for a percentage of the sale. What else do you own of value? I sold the name of my business to an organization that had been using it illegally. That revenue carried us for several months.

**Save money by cancelling obligations.** Health club memberships, vehicle leases, subscriptions: look for ways to have them cancelled, suspended, or reduced. Call and ask: you may run into a reasonable, compassionate human being who knows how to work the system to your benefit.

**Ask young-adult family members to step up to the plate.** If you have teenagers at home, ask them what they can do to help. They may surprise you! Anything they can do will build their character, providing it does not interfere with their studies. The same goes for college students, too.

**Consider debt-counseling services.** If you do not have the financial or emotional wherewithal for the above strategies, look into debt-counseling services, preferably a nonprofit one that will not charge a fee. You don't need to incur more debt while attempting to manage debt! (I cannot vouch for debt counseling services, however, as I have never used one.)



**Deal with debt as soon as you can.** In a health crisis, the trauma of debt can be hard to face. But there is life after the hospital, and the sooner you can deal with the financial aftermath, the more likely you can get it under control. You might even find, as I did, that money matters can be a welcome distraction, even during the illness. With these issues I could actually accomplish some tasks, even when all else was out of my control. And the finances are always part of the journey.

## Understanding Hospital Bills: Tips for Advocates

Tons of mistakes are made on hospital bills—mistakes you will ultimately pay for if you fail to exercise close oversight. And we are indeed responsible for payment. Among the patient responsibilities in the Patient Advocacy Statement is this one: *Meet financial commitments by promptly meeting any financial obligation agreed to with the hospital.* But let's protect our rights while meeting this responsibility. We can insist on satisfactory documentation directly from our providers, and clear explanations from our insurers. This process will inevitably give you gastrointestinal problems, but the pain can be minimized with some preparation.

Every hospital, and every insurance carrier, has its own accounting procedures and paperwork templates. Let's look at one example—an actual statement for Bill's medical expenses—and walk through it step by step. That's how carefully you'll need to review every bill and statement you receive, too.

| HOSPITAL NAME<br>HOSPITAL CONTACT INFO | | STATEMENT DATE<br>ACCOUNT NO.<br>PATIENT NAME<br>MEDICAL RECORD NO.<br>AMOUNT DUE | |
|---|---|---|---|
| **MO/DY/YR** | **Provider/Description of Services** | **Billed to Insurance** | **Personal Balance** |
| | The following services were provided by:<br>NAME OF DOCTOR | | |
| 1/13/2001 | PLACEMENT OF DRAINS, PERI 1 | | 770.00 3 |
| 1/13/2001 | ARTERIAL LINE PERCUTANEOUS | | 225.00 3 |
| 1/13/2001 | INSERT CENT VEN CATH PERC | | 251.00 3 |
| 1/13/2001 | BLOOD GASES | | 250.00 3 |
| 1/13/2001 | ANESTHESIA COMP BY EMERGE | | 110.00 3 |
| 2/20/2001 | PMT–Name of Insurance Co. | | -456.20 4 |
| 2/20/2001 | ADJUSTMENT | | -1065.75 5 |
| 3/09/2001 | PMT ON ACCT/AUTO CBO CHEC | | -114.05 6 |
| 4/03/2001 | INSERT CENT VEN CATH PERC 2 | 251.00 2 | |
| 6/27/2001 | UNLISTED PROCEDURE, VASC | 330.00 7 | |

Steps in billing (numbers correspond with steps):

1. Hospital/Doctor provides service (you will get separate invoices from both, which can be confusing).
2. Hospital/Doctor bills insurance company for service. Amount is placed in "Billed to Insurance" column.
3. At some point, the Hospital/Doctor determines that the Insurance Company has either paid all it is going to pay or, in the absence of any payment, that the patient is responsible for the entire amount. The fee for the service then moves to the "Personal Balance" column.
4. Insurance Company pays and sends an Explanation of Benefits (EOB) to Hospital/Doctor and Patient ("the Insured").
5. Insurance Company deducts a certain amount, based on any previous "Preferred Provider" agreement it has made with the Hospital/Doctor.
6. Unknown payment to account.
7. Unknown procedure done that may, justifiably, result in refusal to pay by Insurance Company.

Without even considering the ethics of the billing system, let's look at what is wrong with this bill, in practical terms, step by step (number by number).

1. The name of the service provided is abbreviated and/or in jargon laypeople rarely understand.
2. The charge billed to the insurance company is often positioned nowhere close to the actual charge on the bill: sometimes it's on a different page. As a result, you have to hunt and crosscheck to ensure all charges have been submitted to the insurance company.
3. Apparently, the first five items here had previously been submitted to the insurance company for payment. But I cannot be sure unless I check prior bills from this provider and look for the same charges in the "Billed to Insurance" column. In any case, I don't know:
    a. Has the provider actually received a Determination of Benefits statement from my insurance carrier? (I don't know unless I can match this bill up with the carrier's Explanation of Benefits statement.)
    b. Or has the provider simply decided the insurance company has had enough time to process this change, and is now moving on to attempt full collection from the patient?
4. The minus sign shows that the provider actually did receive money from the insurance company. But what was the payment for? To find out, I'd have to match this credit up with a payment listed on the Explanation of Benefits statement from the insurance company. But even then, it's tricky: the EOB usually lists multiple charges, and the provider may have added up several of them for this payment, making it all but impossible to know which ones are involved.
5. This is an amount of money the hospital will never collect, and they "write it off" as the cost of participating in this insurance carrier's plan. Again, there may be multiples.
6. Who made the payment under this entry? I am clueless, as apparently is the provider. It wasn't from us—"the Insured"—but far be it from me to

dispute any credit! Note, however, that this credit might be removed at some future time, and since you don't know where the money came from, you can't dispute its removal.

7. This is sure to be an insurance collection problem because the specific nature of the procedure was not described ("coded") correctly. All we know is that some sort of vascular-related procedure was done. Without the specifics, the insurance company will deny benefits. (In this case, rather than correct the coding, this provider moved the charge to the "Personal Balance" column in a subsequent bill and sent it to an outside collection agency, which harassed us for payment. )



A further note on collection agencies: one such agency told us that providers are often more willing to supply documentation than the patient or insurance company is—because they want their money! What is wrong with this picture? Bill and I were ultimately pursued by five collection agencies—one for as little as $84—because the documentation was either erroneous or not forthcoming. This after our respective insurance companies had paid out some $1.75 million in claims!

In sum: ask questions, insist on documentation, and negotiate. You need not feel daunted by the complexity of the paperwork. Take it a step at a time, dealing with issues as they arise. Remember these two points:

- Challenge anything that does not look right to you! Ask for clarification and more documentation. You have the right to require the hospital to detail every expense associated with every service. Make the providers and insurance carriers live up to their obligations
- Get help with these financial matters if you do not wish to spend your energy on it. Help is available from many sources.

One final note: Save all your statements and light a bonfire when you are absolutely certain that all your medical payments are behind you. And most of all, remember: you are not alone!

AFTERWORD

# LIFE AND SPIRIT: THE NEXT SIX YEARS

*The problem is . . . that we are unwilling to give up those things we wish were true. Knowledge is awareness of the parts, wisdom is understanding how those parts work together. This is why a smart man manipulates the parts, while a wise man succumbs to the ministrations of the whole.*

— JESSE WOLF HARDIN, *The Canyon Testament*

For us, our birth is an arrival on this plane, at this time. For our parents, our birth is not only a blessed arrival, it is also a departure: it represents the end of the "one-on-oneness" a mother feels for her unborn child, the end of a previous stage of life for father and mother. With this birth comes a loss, the knowledge that things will be different from now on. Thus the conundrum of life begins.

My own life has always been entwined with death—a conundrum that has taken me years to resolve, to see as part of a larger whole, a pattern of healing.

My childhood was filled with shadows. When I was fifteen, my father died suddenly and, over the next four years, I quickly took on adult responsibilities. I essentially raised my younger sister and cared for our mother, who had descended into a deep depression. I managed the finances and family transportation. And, as I grew up ahead of schedule, the shadows always seemed to hover nearby: I lost three grandparents, then my beloved dog, then my best friend, then the first man I ever loved.

"Knowledge is awareness of the parts," says Jesse Hardin, and for me, knowledge came slowly—let alone wisdom. I was all too aware of my losses, but I did not yet realize that they were forging me as nothing else could have done. I wanted the normal life that had been denied me, preferably one with a fairy-tale ending: ". . . those things we wish were true." So I spent many years wearing an invisible veil, fearing more loss, afraid to look left or right, never letting others glimpse me, my true self. When I met Bill, I discovered a man who, for his own reasons, could not or would not squarely face the idea of death: thus, ours was a match made by a common aversion. Only later did I realize that by running away from the idea of death, we became a powerful magnet for it.

Despite this fact—indeed, barely aware of it—Bill and I built a happy life together. We grew our family by adding four-leggeds, blending our hobbies, sharing our passions, and loving each other.

One evening in September of 2000, Bill called me to the back door of our home in a hushed voice. Staring back at us from our fence railing was a barred owl. The owl was looking straight at us from the deck railing in that unnerving, unblinking manner. This appearance frightened me. I knew that in many Native American traditions, owls represent death—and here it had presented itself to my husband.

One month after we saw the barred owl, Bill was admitted to the hospital with acute pancreatitis, a life-threatening disease. Talk about a wake-up call! No more veil for this gal! Death had come calling in a loud voice and, whether it was invited or not, I *had* to listen. Slowly, I began to get it. Through Bill's illness, I would be the one who would witness to his whole being, who would see to the "ministrations of the whole."

Many of the doctors who treated my husband were specialists, trained to focus on specific body parts. This seemed fine at first, but then Bill suffered multiple organ dysfunction syndrome: just about every part of his body failed, virtually at the same time. Each drug administered to help one part of his body had an adverse impact on other parts. Had I lost him at that point, his autopsy report could easily have read "Death by specialty." No one had been watching the whole patient. I started to see that "Knowledge is awareness of the parts, wisdom is understanding how those parts work together."

To say that I now understood the reason for my lifelong dances with death would not be true. What I can say is that I realized I was no longer an impotent teenager, and I was sick and tired of losing my loved ones. Bill's journey to death's door didn't guarantee his crossing, and I had a role to play.

---

Even before Bill's illness, I was slowly realizing that the series of losses and burdens in my life was preparing me for something. In fact, I was becoming a healer; I was being initiated into shamanism. Such an initiation often entails death and rebirth: in this way shamans are often called to their role.

Most of us never understand the call while in process. It is only when we begin to discover and follow our own spiritual path that we are drawn to a world where everything is connected, where death "births" a new state of being, where our work embraces the journey to the other side, whether in healthcare, ministry, or just plain being. I found my way to shamanism through a series of coincidences that brought me face to face with others who had experienced the same type and extent of loss—and yet they displayed beauty, peace, and grace in their lives. That beauty, peace, and grace was compelling for me, so I followed, and through training and an apprenticeship, learned how to achieve it for myself and share it with others as a part of a worldwide community of healers.

It took months to define my role with Bill, but in retrospect, I can now identify some of the healing techniques I intuitively used. I see them falling within the parameters of the shamanic concept of soul retrieval, because I believe that soul loss is one way to describe Bill's illness.

In most indigenous cultures, healing requires treatment of the body, mind, and soul as a whole. Health is a state of harmony with the self and others. Western medicine is primarily based on the scientific method, which holds the intellect—the mind—as the only tool at our disposal. "Getting up in the head" at the disadvantage of the feet and the soul is part of modern "dis-ease" today and creates stress, rather than harmony, balance, and functionality. Only recently have Westerners woken up to the power of energy-based healing techniques to restore this natural state: traditions such as shamanism, Tai Chi, and Reiki. Soul retrieval, then, is part of healing and represents one method to "welcome home" lost parts of our soul.

What is soul loss? As teacher and author Sandra Ingerman describes it, when we undergo an emotional or physical trauma, a piece of our spiritual body departs in order to survive. "While this is a brilliant survival technique and enables us to deal with pain and loss, when soul loss occurs, that departed piece of our spiritual body doesn't come back on its own."[1] Common causes of soul loss include "abuse, surgery, accidents, war, natural disaster, and addictions." And what are its symptoms? "Dissociation, defined as when we are 'not present' in our body, post-traumatic stress syndrome, addictions, including 'wanting more,' chronic illness, chronic depression or suicide tendencies, grief that never ends," says Ingerman, adding that in a coma, more of the soul is outside the body than inside the body. When you hear someone say, "I've never been the same since . . ." in a negative way, that could be a sign of soul loss.

In its purest form, soul retrieval involves a ceremony in which a shamanic practitioner uses drumming to enter a deep state of meditation on behalf of a friend, family member, colleague, or someone who comes in need. Ceremony or ritual is employed because it creates the power to change. We conduct a "journey" in which we commune with the person's spirit and attempt to discover what has been lost, returning it to the spirits who can then decide whether to return the lost part to the person. In this way, we keep our ego out of the way. We seek assistance from ancestors, power animals, and spirit, all for the greater good—a broad view that requires us to detach emotionally from the outcome.

Ingerman offers us the following wisdom in her teachings—paraphrased here in italics by me, and followed with my comments on how I applied these ideas as Bill's patient advocate.

---

1 Sandra Ingerman's comments, paraphrased here unless otherwise cited, were made during her Soul Retrieval workshop, Sept. 21–26, 2003, attended by the author.

*All healing is done by creating space from the heart. Spirits can only work through the heart. They are the healers.*

As noted earlier, Ingerman has also said it this way: "It is only love that heals. Techniques don't heal. Where there is an open heart there is the energy to bring through miraculous and magical energy. Love is the great transformer."[2] I only knew how to help my husband through my heart, through my love. I used that love to take notes and ask questions, to challenge and push back, to prove myself a partner with Bill's care providers.

*Anxiety occurs when you are in a state separate from spirit. If you can't get emotionally detached, you can't let spirit through.*

I was in a state of constant terror for the first few weeks of Bill's illness. I discovered that I could not communicate with spirit while in this state. In this state, I could only seek what I wanted. The answer, for me, was grounding. One day while I was in one of these frenzied states in the hospital, a friend suggested I go outside, remove my shoes and socks, and stand on the grass. I was to take three deep breaths and, upon each exhalation, send my fear down into the earth. I did so, even with a dusting of snow on the ground, and it helped—so I did it repeatedly throughout Bill's hospitalization. This action enabled me to communicate with spirit, both Bill's and the universe's, as a whole and get out of the way of the outcome.

*Have the client bring some favorite items to the ceremony.*

Since Bill was unconscious and could not choose his favorite things, I did it for him. These included pictures of our dogs, model trains that he enjoyed, and magazines. I also brought photographs of him happy and healthy, and posted them in his room.

2 Sandra Ingerman, *Medicine for the Earth.*

*Symptoms of soul loss include coma, where more of the soul is outside the body than inside. When working with a client in a coma, ask the spirits if they are trying to get out or come back in, and ask what the ethical action is in this situation.*

During two of Bill's septic episodes, he was placed in a medically induced coma. I sat with his hand in mine, telling him, "If you have to go, I will try to understand. I will support your choice. However, I don't want you to go. I need you. Please stay with me." In this case, I was talking directly to Bill's spirit—and I actually felt him come back.

*Shamanic art does not represent power, it is power.*

During a visit to Bill's hospital room, a friend of mine described a protective angel that she saw sitting at the head of the bed. She brought a drawing of it with her on her next visit. That angel was posted on the wall facing Bill's bed, and the drawing followed him around from hospital to hospital. Upon his release, we placed her in our bedroom. Bill named her his "healing angel." God comes in many forms.

*When calling in the spirits, set your intention. Otherwise it's like placing a phone call and then saying nothing. Eventually, the other party hangs up! Intention creates action and allows miracles. Another translation of Jesus's words "Heal in my name" is "Know God and heal as God does." Union with the creative life force is essential to true healing.*

I am a deeply spiritual person, but I would not say that I am religious. I prayed to whatever higher power would listen. I asked for "healing for Bill's highest good," a phrase taught to me by a dear friend who performed Reiki on Bill daily for three months. I asked others to pray, and they did. Our prayers were answered with Bill's survival.

*Traditionally, shamans were also psychological consultants who told healing stories. A story can curse a person, or help heal. Words are like seeds. If you plant seeds of fear, you get fear. People in our culture need hope, inspiration, and love.*

When Bill was in his most critically ill state, a well-meaning friend suggested that I face the likelihood that Bill would not make it, and that I would be alone.

I told my friend that my job today was to do all I could to help Bill stay alive—as long as he wanted to remain here—and that I would face that problem if and when it happened.



*If you go to the future and get bad news, the spirits are showing you this because it can be changed. Quantum physics tells us that the observer changes the observed.*

After incurring some brain damage, Bill mentioned that there was a skinny little man under my bed who blew on an empty pop bottle during the night, and it was frightening him. This vision of the future was terrifying for both of us, and I was determined to debunk it. I lifted up my chair bed and showed him the perfectly normal underside. Bill calmed and returned to sleep without drugs; soon his mind began to heal. Caroline Casey, an American astrologer, says, "Imagination lays the tracks for the reality train to drive down." With our imagination, we have the ability to create our universe.

*Bring friends or family, because soul loss comes from isolation. Allow community to . . . welcome them back.*

At first I actually had to stop the flow of visitors to Bill's room because, I thought, it was wearing *me* out. True, but today, I also believe that the visits weren't what Bill needed just then: in fact, he had not yet decided to remain on this plane. Even in his unconscious state, the visits upset him and he needed help to calm down. But later, visitors were welcome—even our four dogs, thanks to a few tolerant nurses. Later, hundreds of guests came to his welcome-home party. Clearly, Bill had decided to stay.

---

To a shaman, the soul is the place of life's breath, where essence resides, and any physical illness is inextricably linked with it. Illness may be caused by partial soul loss; total soul loss results in death.

Had Bill been losing parts of his soul? Louise Hay identifies the cause of pancreatitis as a "loss of the sweetness of life."[3] This certainly fit Bill. Before

3 Louise Hay, *Heal Your Body A–Z* (Carlsbad, CA: Hay House, 1998).

his illness, he had become increasingly despondent about his work; it was becoming clear that he would not receive the recognition he both craved and deserved. Today, Bill's work is to rediscover that sweetness. This is his version of Soul Remembering, trying to understand and recapture the original beauty of his life. We all need to know our adventures, gifts, and talents. I know that is why he is still here—his work is not done.

Nor is mine. Ingerman believes that "in shamanism, the spirits pick you to do the work. We get initiated into this work. Through initiation, you lose everything in life in order to keep your heart open. Seeing in shamanism is seeing with your heart." To finally go into death, for me, has been a rebirth. To redefine death not as a termination point but as a transition to the next plane: that has given me a wonderful vision of my future, whether near or far away. I recently helped my stepfather cross over, something I probably could not have done with Bill, who had my heart.

My heart undoubtedly got in the way of my spiritual neutrality regarding Bill's survival. Perhaps the strength of my want and need kept him here when he should have crossed. I will never know. I do know, however, that death is no longer a conundrum for me. I have arrived at my life's work through death's door. And of course I will depart through that door as well.

We all intuitively want stories to have a happy ending. Ours does, although not in the way one might wish. Bill and I are no longer together. We divorced in 2006 in the spring, not coincidentally the season of rebirth.

"My Husband Survived, But the Man I Married Didn't," was the title of a newspaper article I read around that time. In part, this describes what happened to us. Bill's brain damage dramatically changed him, and he is very aware of these changes. He fights and resists most of them, and I was present for years of his anger and frustration. It is my belief that in order to create a new reality in a new environment, we must be able to see the beauty in all things. To see that beauty, we must live in a state of appreciation and gratefulness. Bill does not yet live there. Most people drawn to shamanism are empaths, but perhaps I took on pain that was not mine.

I also know that my caregiving, coupled with my terror, stress, and exhaustion, dramatically changed me. Peter Dickinson described my situation well:

"*. . . betrayed by happenings beyond her sphere, and now she was expected to live and behave like a normal citizen, despite that.*"[4] Moreover, I did not follow my own advice. I did not take care of myself. During the six years after Bill's discharge, I gained weight and suffered from borderline diabetes, high blood pressure, and depression—and I seemed caught in my own poor self-care. Since I could change neither Bill's behavior nor, seemingly, my own, I knew that if I did not leave, I would die. I had to "give up those things we wish were true."

So I left, still filled with love for my husband and deep appreciation for his pain and suffering. It was truly the hardest thing I have ever done, harder than the seven months of hell in the hospital, harder than the six years of his subsequent anger, harder than all the deaths that had gone before. But my death would serve no one.

Bill does not understand my choice. I don't believe he ever will. There are days when I have to remind myself why I chose to leave, days when I am lonely or anxious about finances and the future. However, every once in awhile, I find myself smiling. I feel joy in the most unexpected ways. I have come back to myself, something I was unable to do while with Bill—who, I believed, needed everything I had to give to stay alive.

As Ingerman points out, "It is who we become that changes the world, not what we do." And I had to, once again, become myself. The mistake I made was to give everything to Bill and keep nothing for myself. Apparently, this is one of the lessons I am here to learn: that I am important in my own right, and that suicide in service to another is not service, it is suicide.

In Rachel Naomi Remen's words, "To serve is to make whole in some way. . . It's more of a grace. It's very close to love, but a very pure kind of love. A befriending of the life in others, unconditionally."[5] My advocacy supported Bill's return to the wholeness of life, albeit without some of the parts. Neither I nor anyone else can make him as whole as he was before his illness. And that is the rub for him.

---

4 Peter Dickinson, *Some Deaths Before Dying* (New York: Warner Books/Mysterious Press, 1999), 189.

5 Rachel Naomi Remen, interviewed by Peter Marshall, "The Doctor's Dilemma," *Whole Earth Magazine,* Summer 2000.

I still have hope—hope that some day we can find our way back to each other. And there I live, even up to this day.

Blessings.

Jari Holland Buck
September 2007

# ACKNOWLEDGMENTS

I gratefully acknowledge the following healthcare providers, friends, and family who played a crucial role in the care and feeding (in the truest sense of the word) of my husband's body and my spirit.

Dorothy Buck
Rebecca Davis, RN
Gigi Fergus, RN
Sandy Ferguson, RN
Ruth Theis, RN
Tim Malloy, RN
Lee Gorcos, RRT
Pam Sagoo, RRT
My friend, Jean, Reiki Practitioner
Mitzi McFatrich, Cranial Sacral Specialist
Randal Brown, MD
Richard Huseman, MD
Larry Botts, MD
James H. Thomas, MD, RVT
Ben Cowley, MD
Franz Winklhofer, MD
Steve Simpson, MD

Ira Silverman, MD
Holly Fritch Kirby, MD
Jane Murray, MD
Pat Bates, MSL, CCC, SLP
Skip Fannen, JD
Susan, Ronald, Jason, and Jeffrey Miller
Janice Ubben
Pat Nasko Smith
Kevin Kelly
Carin Goodemote
Steve Smith
Curt Starnes, JD
Len Chmelka
The Employees of Universal Underwriters Group
The Prayer Circle—Country Club United Methodist Church

I also gratefully acknowledge these sources for reprint permissions.

Pages xxvii, 74, and 120: Quotations from *Awaken to the Healer Within* by Rich Work with Ann Marie Groth (Mosini, WI: Asini Publishing, 1995) are reprinted with permission.

Page 85: FACES Pain Rating Scale from M.J. Hockenberry, D. Wilson, and M.L. Winkelstein, Wong's *Essentials of Pediatric Nursing*, ed. 7 (St. Louis, 2005), page 1259, used with permission. Copyright Mosby.

Pages 124–126: "Ten Warning Signs of Caregiver Stress" reprinted with permission of the Alzheimer's Association.

Pages 131 and 150: Quotations © Clarissa Pinkola Estés, PhD. All rights reserved. Printed here by kind permission of author and publisher. For permission to reprint: Ngandelman@aol.com

Pages 134–136: "A Consumer Fact Sheet: The Role of the Patient Advocate" reprinted with permission of the National Patient Safety Foundation © NPSF 2003.

Pages 143: Quotations in "Laying the Groundwork for Effective Negotiation" reprinted with permission from Benyus, Janine M., *Biomimicry: Innovation Inspired by Nature* (New York: William Morrow, 1997), copyrighted by Janine M. Benyus.

Pages 163–164: "The Fearless Caregiver Manifesto," from *How to Get the Best Care for Your Loved One and Still Have a Life of Your Own* by Gary Barg, editor and publisher of *Today's Caregiver Magazine* and caregiver.com, reprinted with permission.

Pages 177–179: Sandra Ingerman's text and paraphrased quotations, as cited, reprinted with permission.

Appendix A

# PATIENT FORMS

- Sample *Durable Medical Power of Attorney* Form
- Sample *Living Will* Form
- Sample *Out-of-Hospital "Do Not Resuscitate" Order*
- Instructions for First Responders/EMS
- Sample *Anatomical Gifts* Form
- Sample *Power of Attorney* Form
- Sample *HIPAA Waiver*

## Sample *Durable Medical Power of Attorney* Form

**EXAMPLE ONLY. DO NOT COPY.**
**Each state has different requirements.**
**Consult with a legal advisor for access to documents appropriate for your state.**

State of ______________________
County of ___________________________
This *POWER OF ATTORNEY* is made on (date) ____________________.

I, (name) __________________, of (street address) __________________, (city) ______________, (county) ______________________, (state) _________ (zip) ___________, appoint (spouse or other party) ________________, of (street address) ______________________, (city) __________________, (county) _______________________, (state) _____ (zip) _________, as my attorney-in-fact to act for me, and in my name in any way I could act in person, to make any and all decisions for me concerning my personal care, medical treatment, hospitalization and healthcare in accordance with the terms of this *Durable Power of Attorney.*

Attorney-in-fact is granted authority to require, withhold or withdraw any type of medical treatment or procedure, in accordance with the terms of this durable *Power of Attorney*, even though my death may ensue. Attorney-in-fact shall have the same access to my judicial records that I would have if I were in full health, including the right to disclose the contents to others. Attorney-in-fact shall also have full power to make a disposition of any part or all of my body for medical purposes, to authorize an autopsy and to direct the disposition of my remains.

The above grant of power is intended to be a broad as possible so that attorney-in-fact will have authority to make any decision I could make to obtain or terminate any type of healthcare, including withdrawal of food and water and other life-sustaining measures if attorney-in-fact believes such action would be consistent with my intent and desires.

This *Power of Attorney* shall become effective on [date]. This *Power of Attorney* shall terminate upon a written revocation by [name] or by a court of competent jurisdiction.

If any attorney-in-fact named by me shall die, become legally disabled, resign, refuse to act or be unavailable, I name the following persons, each to act alone and successively in the order named, as successors to attorney-in-fact: (different party than above) ______________, (street address) _____________, (city) __________________, (county) ______________, (state) _______ (zip) __________,

If a guardian of my person is to be appointed, I nominate the following person to serve as guardian: (spouse or other party) _______________, of (address) _________________, (city) _____________, (county) ___________, (state) _____ (zip) ____________,

I am fully informed as to all of the contents of this form and understand the full import of this grant of powers to my attorney-in-fact.

___________________________________ ___________________________________
(name) (date)

## Sample *Living Will* Form

**EXAMPLE ONLY. DO NOT COPY.**
**Each state has different requirements.**
**Consult with a legal advisor for access to documents appropriate for your state.**

DECLARATION IN CONFORMANCE
WITH [state] STATUTES [number/s]

I have the primary right to make my own decisions concerning treatment that might unduly prolong the dying process. By this declaration I express to my physician, family and friends my intent. If I should have a terminal condition, it is my desire my dying not be prolonged by administration of death-prolonging procedures. If my condition is terminal and I am unable to participate in decisions regarding my medical treatment, I direct that my attending physician withhold or withdraw medical procedures that merely prolong the dying process and are not necessary to my comfort or to alleviate pain. It is not my intent to authorize affirmative or deliberate acts or omissions to shorten my life, rather, only to permit the natural process of dying.

____________________________ ____________________________

(name) (date)

City of residence: ____________________________
County of residence: ____________________________
State of residence: ____________________________

The declarant is known to me, is eighteen years of age or older, of sound mind, and voluntarily signed this document in my presence.

Witness ____________________________
Address: ____________________________

Witness ____________________________
Address: ____________________________

## Sample *Out-of-Hospital "Do Not Resuscitate" Order*

**EXAMPLE ONLY. DO NOT COPY.**
**Each state has different requirements.**[1]
**Consult with a legal advisor for access to documents appropriate for your state.**

| DO NOT RESUSCITATE |
|---|

**ALL FIRST RESPONDERS AND EMERGENCY MEDICAL SERVICES PERSONNEL ARE AUTHORIZED TO COMPLY WITH THIS *OUT-OF-HOSPITAL DNR ORDER*.**

This request for no resuscitative attempts in the event of a cardiac and/or respiratory arrest for: ______________________________, has been ordered by the
PLEASE PRINT NAME
physician whose signature appears below. This *Order* is in compliance with the patient's/surrogate's wishes and it has been determined and documented by the physician below that resuscitation attempts for this patient would be medically inappropriate.

It is expected that this *DNR Order* shall be honored by all Emergency Medical Services (EMS) personnel, First Responders and other healthcare providers who may have contact with this patient during a medical emergency.

PATIENT/SURROGATE SIGNATURE ______________________
PATIENT'S ADDRESS ______________________

**<u>THE ABOVE-NAMED PATIENT IS UNDER THE CARE OF:</u>**

PHYSICIAN NAME ______________________
PLEASE PRINT NAME
PHYSICIAN ADDRESS ______________________
TELEPHONE NUMBER ______________________
MEDICAL FACILITY AFFILIATION ______________________
PHYSICIAN SIGNATURE ______________________

**THIS DOCUMENT SHOULD BE PROMINENTLY DISPLAYED AND READILY AVAILABLE TO EMS PERSONNEL**
**(see reverse for instructions)**



1 This form adapted from American College of Emergency Physicians, New Jersey Chapter, "New Jersey Do Not Resuscitate (DNR) Orders," Medical Society of New Jersey, August 2003, http://www.msnj.org/Resources/Reports/DNRGuidelines.pdf.

## Instructions for First Responders/EMS

All patients have the right to make healthcare decisions including the right to accept or refuse life-saving medical treatment.

1. Assess the patient for the absence of breathing and/or heartbeat.
2. If the patient *is not* in cardiac and/or respiratory arrest, provide all necessary care including transport if required.
3. If the patient *is* in cardiac and/or respiratory arrest, *do not initiate* CPR and resuscitative efforts.
4. Follow local EMS protocols for pronouncement.
5. Document all pertinent information on your run sheet and attach a copy of the *out-of-hospital DNR order*.
6. *Only* the designated individual(s) (patient, surrogate or physician) who signed this form may rescind it at any time.
7. Photocopies of this document *are permitted* and shall be honored at all times.

This document, its intent and associated policies are supported by:

Medical Society of [sample state]
[Sample state] Department of Health and Senior Services
Office of EMS
American College of Physicians, [Sample state] Chapter
[Sample state] Nurses Association
[Sample state] Health Decisions
[Sample state] Hospice and Palliative Care Association
Academy of Medicine of [Sample state]
[Sample state] MICU Advisory Council
[Sample state] First Aid Council
Office of the Ombudsman for the Institutionalized Elderly
[Sample state] Hospital Association

IF THERE ARE ANY QUESTIONS REGARDING THE TREATMENT OR PRONOUNCEMENT OF THIS PATIENT, CALL:

CONTACT PERSON ________________________________
TELEPHONE NUMBER ______________________________
AGENCY ______________________________________

## Sample *Anatomical Gifts* Form

**EXAMPLE ONLY. DO NOT COPY.**
**Each state has different requirements.**[2]
**Consult with a legal advisor for access to documents appropriate for your state.**

Pursuant to the provisions of the Uniform Anatomical Gift Act, Article #X of the [sample state] Public Health Code, I hereby give my whole body, to be delivered after my death as provided in the aforementioned law, to the Anatomical Donations Program of the University of [sample state] Medical School to be used in medical education and research. I also permit use of my medical information by the Anatomical Donations Program.

I have checked those statements below that apply to my intended donation.

- ❑ My body may be used in any manner that the University of [sample state] Medical School deems necessary.
- ❑ Part or all of my body may be permanently preserved for teaching purposes.
- ❑ I am registered with an organ/tissue donation agency (see Organ Donation).

Has a relative donated to the Anatomical Donations Program before? Yes No
Name of Relative: ______________________________

Send one signed and witnessed copy of this form to: Anatomical Donations Program, The University of [sample state] Medical School, [sample address]. Keep a copy of this form for your records.



______________________________
Print Donor Name

______________________________
Donor Signature

______________________________
______________________________
Print Donor Address

______________________________
Donor Date of Birth

______________________________
______________________________
Witnesses (2 required)

______________________________
Date Signed

(_____) ______________________________
Donor Telephone Number

---

2 This form adapted from University of Michigan Health System, "Gift of Human Anatomy to the University of Michigan," http://www.med.umich.edu/anatomy/donors/print_form.html.

## Sample *Power of Attorney* Form

**EXAMPLE ONLY. DO NOT COPY.**
**Each state has different requirements.**
**Consult with a legal advisor for access to documents appropriate for your state.**

KNOW ALL MEN BY THESE PRESENTS:
(name) ________________________________, hereinafter referred to as PRINCIPAL, in the County of ______________________, State of ___________________________ does appoint (name) ___________________________________ his true and lawful attorney.

In principal's name, and for principal's use and benefit, said attorney is authorized hereby:
(1) To demand, sue for, collect, and receive all money, debts, accounts, legacies, bequests, interest, dividends, annuities, and demands as are now or shall hereafter become due, payable, or belonging to principal, and take all lawful means, for the recovery thereof and to compromise the same and give discharges for the same;

(2) To buy and sell land, make contracts of every kind relative to land, any interest therein or the possession thereof, and to take possession and exercise control over the use thereof;

(3) To lease, buy, sell, mortgage, hypothecate, assign, transfer, and in any manner deal with goods, wares and merchandise, chooses in action, certificates or shares of capital stock, and other property in possession or in action, and to make, do, and transact all and every kind of business of whatever nature;

(4) To execute, acknowledge, and deliver contracts of sale, escrow instructions, deeds, leases including leases for minerals and hydrocarbon substances and assignments of leases, covenants, agreements and assignments of agreements, mortgages and assignments of mortgages, conveyances in trust, to secure indebtedness or other obligations, and assign the beneficial interest thereunder, subordinations of liens or encumbrances, bills of lading, receipts, evidences of debt, releases, bonds, notes, bills, requests to reconvey deeds of trust, partial or full judgments, satisfactions of mortgages, and other debts, and other written instruments of whatever kind and nature, all upon such terms and conditions as said attorney shall approve.

Giving and granting to said attorney full power and authority to do all and every act and thing whatsoever requisite and necessary to be done relative to any of the foregoing as fully to all intents and purposes as principal might or could do if personally present.

All that said attorney shall lawfully do or cause to be done under the authority of this *Power of Attorney* is expressly approved.

______________________________ ______________________________
(name) (date)

## Sample *HIPAA Waiver*

**EXAMPLE ONLY. DO NOT COPY.**
**Each attorney has his/her own personalized *HIPAA Waiver*.**
**Consult your attorney.**

I hereby waive, and any Agent agreeing to serve as Agent hereunder shall be deemed to have waived, any physician-client privilege for the limited purpose of determining the disability or incapacity hereunder of an Agent or myself and authorize the disclosure of such certification by the physician for use by that person as necessary hereunder. All healthcare providers are absolved and released of any liability for providing health information to my Agent. For purposes of the privacy rule of the United States Department of Health and Human Services promulgated pursuant to the Health Insurance Portability & Accountability Act of 1996 (HIPAA) for purposes of determining whether I am incapacitated or disabled, requests for disclosure of health information made by my Agent (regardless of whether it has previously been determined that I am incapacitated or disabled) shall be deemed to be requests for disclosure made by me and disclosures of health information, including a certification as to whether or not I am under a disability or incapacity, to my Agent shall be deemed to be disclosure made to me.

________________________________ ________________________
(name) (date)

City of residence: ______________________________
County of residence: ______________________________
State of residence: ______________________________

The declarant is known to me, is eighteen years of age or older, of sound mind and voluntarily signed this document in my presence.
Witness ______________________________
Address ______________________________

Witness ______________________________
Address ______________________________

Appendix B

# HOSPITAL FORMS

- Sample *Patient Advocacy Statement*
- Sample *Medical Information and Privacy Statement*

## Sample *Patient Advocacy Statement*

**EXAMPLE ONLY. DO NOT COPY.**
**Each hospital has its own personalized *Patient Advocacy Statement.***
**Consult your hospital.**



*Patient Rights*

Quality patient care is the primary concern of [Sample Hospital]'s Health System. You or your designated representative have the right to:

- Treatment without discrimination as to race, age, religion, sex, national origin, disability, or source of payment.
- Considerate and respectful care.
- Receive care in a safe setting free from abuse, harassment, and neglect.
- Be free from restraints or seclusion, imposed as a means of coercion, discipline, convenience, or retaliation by staff.
- Understandable information concerning diagnosis, treatment and prognosis, and financial implications of treatment choices.
- The identity of those involved in your care.
- Involvement in medical decision making including refusal of care and treatment, to the extent permitted by law, and to be informed of the medical consequences of refusal.
- Make decisions through *Advance Directives* such a *Living Will* or *Durable Medical Power of Attorney.*
- Appoint a surrogate to make healthcare decisions on your behalf to the extent permitted by law.
- Sensitivity addressing issues related to care at the end of life.
- Privacy.
- Confidentiality of information.

- Reasonable access to review the medical records pertaining to your care, and to receive copies of these records for a reasonable photocopying fee.
- Receive medically appropriate care.
- Knowledge related to business relationships of the provider that might affect care.
- Decline participation in experimental treatments.
- Be informed of hospital policies and resources, such as patient advocates and the ethics committee.
- Access an internal grievance process and appeal to an external agency.
- Expect a family member (or representative) and your physician will be notified of your admission to the hospital, unless you request otherwise.
- Be informed of your rights in writing.
- Unrestricted access to communication, visitors, mail, and telephone calls, unless clinically contraindicated. Any restrictions must be fully explained to the patient.
- The appropriate assessment and management of pain.
- Have your rights protected during research, investigation, and clinical trials involving human subjects.
- Access pastoral care and spiritual services.
- Protective oversight while you are in the hospital.
- Be informed of and participate in treatment decisions and the care-planning process.
- Participate in discharge planning, including being informed of service options that are available and choice of agencies.
- Have personal possessions brought to the hospital reasonably protected.
- Expect a reasonable response to your need/request for assistance in effective communication, regardless of language or disability.

We at [sample hospital] welcome your input concerning the care and treatment provided to you. Information received regarding compliments and concerns are tracked and trended in a confidential computer system. This information assists us in our continuing goal of improving care for you and other future patients and customers.

*Patient Compliments*

Our primary goal at [sample hospital] is to make your stay as pleasant as possible. Compliments are welcome and will be shared with the [sample hospital] staff involved.

*Patient Concerns*

Most patient concerns can be handled by [sample hospital] associates at the time the concern is raised. [Sample hospital] associates are encouraged to resolve concerns to the best of their ability with the resources at hand.

In addition, the Patient Advocate Department serves as a liaison between patients, their families, and the hospital. The patient advocate transcends departmental lines and interacts with staff at all levels within the organization.

To reach the patient advocate while you are in the hospital please call ext. XXXX, or (outside direct dial number) from outside the hospital. The patient advocate is available between the hours of X:XX a.m.–X:XX p.m. Monday through Friday.

After hours, weekends, and holidays, assistance may be obtained by calling the hospital operator at “0” while in the hospital or (the outside general hospital number) from outside the hospital.

Once your concern is received, we will start investigating the matter within 24 hours.



*Notice of Patient Grievance Procedure*

A patient grievance is a formal written or verbal grievance that is filed by a patient, when a patient issue cannot be resolved promptly by staff present. Exercising your right to the grievance process will not compromise patient care. Confidentiality will be respected at all times. The expectation is that the facility will handle relatively minor changes in a timely manner with the need for a written facility response.

You have the right to lodge a grievance with any state agency directly, regardless of whether you have first used the hospital’s grievance procedure. A list of state advocacy agencies and phone numbers is provided on the back of this brochure.

### *Patient Responsibilities*

As a patient, you, your family, or your designated representatives have responsibility to:

- Provide information: to the best of your knowledge, accurate and complete information about present complaints, past illnesses, hospitalizations, medications, and other matters relating to your health. The patient and family are responsible for reporting unexpected changes in the patient's condition. The patient and the family help the hospital improve its understanding of the patient's environment by providing feedback about service needs and expectations.
- Report pain: inform care providers of your level of pain and the effectiveness of provided treatment. Ask questions when you do not understand what you have been told about your care or what you are expected to do.
- Follow instructions: you are responsible for following the care, service, or treatment plan developed. You should express any concerns you have about your ability to follow and comply with the proposed care plan or course of treatment. Every effort is made to adapt the plan to your specific needs and limitations. When such adaptations to the treatment plan are not recommended, you and your family are responsible for understanding the consequences of the treatment alternatives and not following the proposed course.
- Accept consequences: you and your family are responsible for the outcomes if you do not follow the care, service or treatment plan.
- Follow rules and regulations: you and your family are responsible for following the hospital's rules and regulations concerning patient care and conduct.
- Show respect and consideration: for the hospital's personnel and property, other patients, help control noise and disturbances, and following smoking policies.
- Meet financial commitments: by promptly meeting any financial obligation agreed to with the hospital.

The patient's family or surrogate decision maker assumes the above responsibility for the patient if the patient has been found by his or her physician to be incapable of understanding these responsibilities, has been judged incompetent in accordance with law, or exhibits a communication barrier.

## Sample *Medical Information and Privacy Statement*

**EXAMPLE ONLY. DO NOT COPY.**
**Each hospital has its own personalized**
***Medical Information and Privacy Statement.***
**Consult your hospital.**

**This notice describes how medical information about you may be used and disclosed and how you can get access to this information. Please review it carefully.**

This page provides a brief summary of your privacy rights. Please read pages X–X for a full description of your rights. if you need more information, you may call Patient Relations at ext. XXXX.

This notice describes the privacy practices of [sample hospital], Holding Company and associated doctors, jointly known as [sample hospital]. These organizations are allowed to share medical information with each other for treatment, payment, and operational activities. We will use this information in order to provide our patients with complete and comprehensive healthcare services.

### *Our Commitment to You*

We are committed to protecting your medical information. [Sample Hospital] is required by law to keep medical information about you private, to give you this Notice about our privacy practices and to follow the practices outlined in this Notice.

### *How We May Use and Disclose Your Medical Information*

We may use your medical information for treatment (such as sending medical information about you to your referring physician), payment (such as sending a bill to your insurance company), and healthcare operations (such as teaching students or evaluating the performance of our staff).

Under certain circumstances we are allowed to use or disclose your medical information without your written permission. We may give out information about you for public health purposes, reports of abuse, neglect, or domestic violence, health oversight audits or inspections, research studies, funeral arrangements and organ donations, government programs, workers' compensation, and emergency situations. We also disclose patient information when required by law, such as in response to a request from law enforcement or in response to judicial orders.

We also may contact you for appointment reminders, to tell you about possible treatment options and health services, or for fundraising efforts. If you are a hospital inpatient, we will put your name in our facility directory unless you tell us otherwise. We may disclose medical information about you to a friend or family member who is involved in your care.

*Your Rights Concerning Your Medical Information*

You have the right to inspect or copy your medical information. There may be a fee for this service. You may ask us to amend the medical information you believe is incorrect or incomplete. You may have a list of non-routine disclosures we have made about you. You may request special confidential communications. You may request restrictions on information disclosed about you. You have the right to complain to us and to the federal government if you believe your privacy rights have been violated. You have a right to a paper copy of this notice.

We reserve the right to make changes to this Notice. We will post a copy of the current Notice in the locations where you receive services.

Effective: [date]

**This notice describes how medical information about you may be used and disclosed and how you can get access to this information. Please review it carefully.**

If you have any questions about this Notice, please call Patient Relations at XXXX.



*Who Will Follow This Notice*

This Notice describes the privacy practices of the [sample hospital]. [Sample hospital] is made up of the separate healthcare organizations listed below. To better serve you, [sample hospital] jointly provides you with this Notice regarding privacy practices of [sample hospital] and your privacy rights established by the Health Insurance Portability and Accountability Act of 1996 (HIPAA). The healthcare organizations that participate in this joint Notice, including their separate sites of services, have each agreed to follow the terms of this Notice as permitted by HIPAA. Upon request, we will provide you with a list of sites and locations of [sample hospital] that apply to this Notice.

The [sample hospital] includes the following organizations:

- The [sample hospital];
- The hospital holding company;
- All of the affiliated doctors.

The organizations listed above include employees, staff, trainees, volunteer groups, and other healthcare personnel.

These organizations, sites and locations may share your medical information with each other for treatment, payment or healthcare operations purposes described in this Notice and are allowed to do so by law for the benefit of providing you with efficient healthcare services.

*Important Disclaimer*

**The organizations participating in this joint notice for [sample hospital] are participating only for the purposes of providing this joint notice and sharing health information as permitted by applicable law and are not in any way providing healthcare services mutually or on each other's behalf. Each organization participating in this joint notice for [sample hospital] is an individual healthcare provider and each is individually responsible for its own activities, including compliance with privacy laws, and all healthcare services it provides.**

*Our Pledge Regarding Medical Information*

We understand that medical information about you and your health is personal. We are committed to protecting medical information about you. We create a record of the care and services you receive at [sample hospital]. We need this record to provide you with complete and comprehensive care and to comply with certain legal requirements. This Notice applies to all of the records your care generates at [sample hospital].

This Notice tells you about the ways in which we may use and disclose medical information about you. It also describes your rights and certain obligations we have regarding the use and disclosure of medical information.

We are required by law to:

- make sure that medical information that identifies you is kept private
- give you this Notice of our legal duties and privacy practices with respect to medical information about you, and
- follow the terms of this Notice currently in effect

***How We May Use and Disclose Medical Information About You***

The following categories describe different ways that we use and disclose medical information. Not every use or disclosure in a category will be listed. However, all of the ways we are permitted to use and disclose information will fall within one of these categories.

1. For Treatment. We may use medical information about you to provide you with medical treatment or services. We may disclose medical information about you to doctors, nurses, technicians, students, or other [sample hospital] personnel. For example, different departments of [sample hospital] may share medical information about you in order to coordinate elements of your care, such as prescriptions, lab work, and X rays. We also may disclose medical information about you to people outside [sample hospital] such as referring physicians and home healthcare nurses in connection with your healthcare treatment.
2. For Payment. We may use and disclose medical information about you to your insurance plan, or other parties who help pay for your care. For example, we may tell your health plan about a treatment you are going to receive to determine whether your plan will pay for that treatment.
3. For Health Care Operations. We may use and disclose medical information about you for [sample hospital] operations. These uses and disclosures are necessary to run [sample hospital] and to make sure that all of our patients receive quality care. For example, we may use medical information to review our treatment and services and to evaluate the performance of our staff in caring for you. We may also disclose information to doctors, nurses, technicians, students, and other healthcare personnel for teaching purposes.

4. Business Associates. There may be some activities provided for our organization through contracts with outside businesses. Examples include transcription services and collection agencies. Under such contracts, we may disclose your health information to these businesses to perform the job we have asked them to do. These contracts also require businesses to protect the health information we disclose to them.

5. Appointment Reminders. We may contact you to remind you about your appointment for medical care.

6. Treatment Alternatives. We may use and disclose medical information to tell you about possible treatment options or alternatives that may be of interest to you and other health-related benefits and services.

7. Hospital Directory. We may include certain limited information about you in the hospital directory while you are an inpatient at the hospital. This information may include your name, location in the hospital, your general condition (fair, stable, etc.), and your religious affiliation. The directory information, except for your religious information, may also be disclosed to people who ask for you by name. Your religious affiliation may be given to a member of the clergy, even if they don't ask for you by name. We provide this service so your family, friends, and clergy can visit you in the hospital and generally know how you are doing. If you are admitted to the hospital, we will not provide this information or even acknowledge your presence in the Hospital at your request. Contact the Admitting Department at XXXX if you do not want this information provided.

8. Individuals Involved in Your Care. Unless you object, we may disclose medical information about you to a friend or family member who is involved in your medical care and we may disclose medical information about you to an entity assisting in a disaster relief effort so that your family can be notified about your location and condition. If you are not present or able to object, then we may, using our professional judgment, determine whether the disclosure is in your best interest.

9. Research. As an academic medical center, we may use and disclose medical information about you for research purposes. We will only use and disclose your

information for a research project if we obtain your permission, or if the need to obtain your permission has been waived by a designated review committee that meets federal requirements.

10. As Required by Law. We will disclose medical information about you when required to do so by federal, state, or local law.

11. Fundraising Activities. We may use information about you to contact you in an effort to raise funds for [sample hospital] and its operations. We may disclose information about you to a foundation related to [sample hospital] so that the foundation may contact you in raising funds, including, for example, mailing you invitations to fundraising events, mailing you annual financial reports, and other types of mailings related to fundraising activities. We would only disclose contact information, such as your name, address and phone number and the dates you received treatment or services. If you do not wish to be contacted for [sample hospital] fundraising purposes, contact [sample hospital] Endowment at ext. XXXX.

12. To Avert a Serious Threat to Health or Safety. We may use and disclose medical information about you when necessary to prevent a serious threat to your health and safety or the health and safety of others. Disclosure would only be to persons who could help prevent the threat.

### *How We May Use and Disclose Medical Information About You– Special Situations*

1. Organ and Tissue Donation. We may disclose medical information to organizations that handle and monitor organ donation and transplantation.

2. Military. If you are a member of the armed forces, we may disclose medical information about you as required by military command authorities. We may also disclose medical information about foreign military personnel to the appropriate foreign military authority.

3. Workers' Compensation. We may disclose medical information about you for workers' compensation or similar programs to the extent necessary to comply with laws relating to workers' compensation or other similar programs established by law. These programs provide benefits for work-related injuries or illness.

4. Public Health Risks. As required by law, we may disclose medical information about you for public health activities. For example, we may undertake these activities:
   a. to prevent or control disease, injury, or disability;
   b. to report births and deaths;
   c. to report child abuse or neglect;
   d. to report reactions to medications or problems with products;
   e. to notify people of recalls of products they may be using;
   f. to notify a person who may have been exposed to a disease or may be at risk for contracting or spreading a disease or condition; and
   g. to notify the appropriate government authority if we believe a patient has been the victim of abuse, neglect, or domestic violence. We will only make this disclosure subject to certain requirements when mandated or authorized by law.
5. Health Oversight Activities and Registries. We may disclose medical information to a health oversight agency for activities authorized by law and to patient registries for conditions such as tumor, trauma, and burn. These oversight activities include, for example, audits, investigations, inspections and licensure surveys. These activities are necessary for the government to monitor the healthcare system, the outbreak of disease, government programs, compliance with civil rights laws, and to improve patient outcomes.
6. Lawsuits and Disputes. If you are involved in a lawsuit or a dispute, we may disclose medical information about you in response to a court or administrative order. We may also disclose medical information about you in response to a subpoena, discovery request, or other lawful process.
7. Law Enforcement. We may disclose medical information if asked to do so by a law enforcement official:
   a. for the reporting of certain types of wounds;
   b. in response to a court order, subpoena, warrant, summons or similar process;
   c. to identify or locate a suspect, fugitive, material witness, or missing person;
   d. about the victim of a crime, if under certain limited circumstances, we are unable to obtain the person's agreement;

e. about a death we believe may be the result of criminal conduct;

f. about suspected criminal conduct on the premises; and

g. in emergency circumstances to report a crime; the location of the crime or victims; or the identity, description, or location of the person who committed the crime.

8. Coroners, Medical Examiners, and Funeral Directors. We may disclose medical information to a coroner or medical examiner. This may be necessary, for example, to identify a deceased person or determine the cause of death. We may also disclose medical information about patients of the hospital to funeral directors as necessary to carry out their duties.

9. National Security. We may disclose medical information about you to authorized federal officials for purposes of national security.

10. Inmates. An inmate does not have the right to this Notice.

*Your Rights Regarding Medical Information About You*

You have the following rights regarding medical information we maintain about you:

1. Right to Inspect and Copy. You have the right to inspect and have copied medical information used to make decisions about your care. Usually, this includes medical and billing records, but does not include some records such as psychotherapy notes. To inspect and have copied medical information used to make decisions about you, you must submit your request in writing. Call Release of Information at XXXX for further details. We may charge a fee for the costs of processing your request. Under very limited circumstances, your request may be denied, such as a request for psychotherapy notes. You may request that a denial be reviewed by contacting Patient Relations at XXXX.

2. Right to Amend. If you feel that medical information we have about you is incorrect or incomplete, you may ask us to amend the information. You have the right to request an amendment of your record for as long as the information is kept by or for [sample hospital]. To request an amendment to your record, your request must be made in writing and submitted to the Director of Medical Records [address]. In

addition, you must provide a reason that supports your request. We may deny your request for an amendment to your record if it is not in writing or does not include a reason to support the request. We also may deny your request if you ask us to amend information that:

a. was not created by us, unless the person or entity that created the information is no longer available to make the amendment

b. is not part of the records used to make decisions about you

c. is not part of the information which you are permitted to inspect and copy, or

d. is accurate and complete

3. Right to an Accounting of Disclosures. You have the right to receive a list of the disclosures we made of your medical information. This list will not include all disclosures made. For example, this list will not include disclosures we made for treatment, payment, healthcare operations, disclosures made prior to [month, day, year], or disclosures you specifically authorized. To request this list or 'account of disclosures', you must submit your request in writing on the authorized form [sample hospital] will provide to you upon request.

4. Right to Request Restrictions. You have the right to request a restriction or limitation on the medical information we use or disclose about you for treatment, payment or healthcare operations. You also have the right to request a limit on the medical information we disclose about you to someone who is involved in your care or in the payment for your care, such as a family member or friend. We are not required to agree to your request. If we do agree, we will comply with your request unless the information is needed to provide you emergency treatment. To request restrictions, you must make your request in writing on a form that will be provided to you, upon your request. You must tell us (1) what information you want to limit, (2) whether you want to limit our use, disclosure, or both, and (3) to whom you want the limits to apply.

5. Right to a Paper Copy of This Notice. You may ask us to give you a copy of this Notice at any time. Even if you have agreed to receive this Notice electronically, you are still entitled to a paper copy of this notice.

### *Revisions to this Notice*

We may revise this Notice to reflect any changes in our privacy practices. We reserve the right to make the revised or changed Notice effective for medical information we already have about you as well as for any information we receive in the future. We will post a copy of the current Notice in the locations where you receive services. The effective date of this notice is found on the first page, in the top right hand corner.

### *Complaints*

If you believe your privacy rights have been violated, you may file a complaint with [Sample Hospital] or with the Secretary of the Department of Health and Human Services. To file a complaint with [Sample Hospital], contact the Privacy Officials of [Sample Hospital], through the office of Patient Relations at ext. XXXX. You will not be penalized for filing a complaint.

### *Other Uses of Medical Information*

Other uses and disclosures of medical information not covered by this Notice or by other laws that apply to us will be made only with your written authorization. If you provide authorization to use or disclose medical information about you, you may revoke that authorization, in writing, at any time. If you revoke your authorization, we will no longer use or disclose medical information about you for the reasons covered by your written authorization. We are unable to take back any disclosures we have already made with your authorization, and we are required to retain records of the care that we provided to you.

# RESOURCES

This resource list has four sections. **General Tools** lists health-related sources of broad interest. In **Resources for Patient Advocates** you will find sources tailored to those of us actively advocating for a loved one. **Palliative Care Resources** lists contacts that are helpful for end-of-life care. In all three sections, quoted passages are the sources' own self-descriptions, often taken directly from their websites. (Note that contact details are accurate as of this book's publication date, but such information often changes.) The last section, **About This Book's Website**, lists some of the resources found at www.hospitalstayhandbook.com. There you may also find additional and updated resource lists for patient advocates.

## General Tools

***Aging with Dignity***

*PO Box 1661*
*Tallahassee, FL 32302-1661*
*Phone: 888-5WISHES (888-594-7437)*
*Fax: 850-681-2481*
*www.agingwithdignity.org/order.html*

This group distributes the Five Wishes document, a type of living will that is legally valid in many U.S. states. It "helps you express how you want to be treated if you are seriously ill and unable to speak for yourself. It is unique among all other living will and health agent forms because it looks to all of a person's needs: medical, personal, emotional and spiritual . . . Five Wishes lets your family and doctors know which person you want to make health care decisions for you when you can't make them, the kind of medical treatment you want or don't want, how comfortable you want to be, how you want people to treat you, and what you want your loved ones to know."

***Caregiver.com***

*Caregiver Media Group*
*3005 Greene Street*
*Hollywood, FL 33020*
*Phone: 800-829-2734*
*Fax: 954-893-1779*
*info@caregiver.com*
*www.caregiver.com*

This website's materials include free e-newsletter subscriptions, an online chat board, and *Caregiver Magazine* articles. The organization also hosts caregiver conferences.

*CaringBridge*

*1995 Rahn Cliff Court, Suite 200*
*Eagan, MN 55122*
*Phone: 651-452-7940*
*Fax: 651-681-7115*
*www.caringbridge.org*

This nonprofit offers "free personalized websites to those wishing to stay in touch with family and friends during significant life events." Their mission is "to bring together a global community of care powered by the love of family and friends in an easy, accessible and private way. CaringBridge authors quickly and easily create personalized websites that display journal entries and photographs. Well-wishers visit the site to read updates and leave messages in the Guestbook."

***Centers for Disease Control and Prevention***

*1600 Clifton Road*
*Atlanta, GA 30333*
*Phone: 800-311-3435*
*www.cdc.gov*

The CDC offers information about existing and emerging diseases, emergency preparedness and response, environmental health, genetics and genomics, health promotion, injury and violence, travelers' health, vaccines and immunizations, and workplace safety and health. The CDC is part of the U.S. Department of Health and Human Services.

***Consumer Reports Best Buy Drugs***

*www.crbestbuydrugs.org*

This site discusses affordable drug treatment options.

### *Discovery Health TV*

*health.discovery.com/encyclopedias/otherdatabases.html*

This site's *Diseases and Conditions Encyclopedia* covers topics such as a nutrition index (eating well, preventing illness, promoting longevity), medical tests (preparing for tests, what to expect, understanding results), surgical procedures (preparation, techniques, recovery, potential complications), and injuries (symptoms, diagnoses, treatments). The site does carry ads.

### *Family Caregiving 101*

*www.familycaregiving101.org*

Sponsored by the National Family Caregivers Association and the National Alliance for Caregiving, this site offers caregivers "the basic tools, skills and information they need to protect their own physical and mental health while they provide high quality care for their loved one. It is also a place for family caregivers to return again and again as new levels of caregiving are reached."

### *Five Criteria for Evaluating Web Pages*

*www.library.cornell.edu/olinuris/ref/research/webcrit.html*

Guidance for finding reliable Internet sources for your research.

### *Health Grades*

*500 Golden Ridge Road, Suite 100*
*Golden, CO 80401*
*Phone: 303-716-0041*
*www.healthgrades.com*

This for-profit group can help you evaluate doctors, hospitals, and nursing homes. For a fee, receive a "report on a specific doctor that includes education, background, board certifications and state/federal disciplinary action." Health Grades reports on "hospital patient safety activities to consumers, payers and employers . . . [and] provides reports to professional medical liability insurance underwriters for nursing homes, hospitals and physicians that assist these companies in assessing risk and verifying background information." Named one of fifty "Most Incredibly Useful Sites" by Yahoo! Internet Life.



***healthfinder***

*PO Box 1133*
*Washington, DC 20013-1133*
*www.healthfinder.gov*

Look here to find the Internet's most reliable government and nonprofit health and human services sources, with links to more than 1,500 carefully selected sites. It also provides relevant gender, age, and ethnicity statistics. The site is a service of the National Health Information Center, U.S. Department of Health and Human Services.

***Health Literacy***

*National Network of Libraries of Medicine*
*National Network Office*
*National Library of Medicine*
*8600 Rockville Pike*
*Building 38, Room B1-E03*
*Bethesda, Maryland 20894*
*http://nnlm.gov/outreach/consumer/hlthlit.html*

"Provides information on health literacy as an important component of health communication, medical product safety and oral health. Sections include: definition, skills needed for health literacy, background, research findings on impact of literacy, economic impact of low health literacy, role of the consumer health librarian, health literacy organizations and programs, bibliographies and webliographies, and health literacy listservs."

***Hospital Compare***

*U.S. Department of Health and Human Services*
*200 Independence Avenue SW*
*Washington, D.C. 20201*
*Phone: 877-696-6775*
*www.hospitalcompare.hhs.gov*

"This website was created through the efforts of the Centers for Medicare & Medicaid Services and the Hospital Quality Alliance. Hospital Compare has quality measures on how often hospitals provide some of the recommended care to get the best results for most patients. You will see some of the recommended care that an adult should get if being treated for a heart attack, heart failure or pneumonia, or having surgery. This information helps you, your health care provider, family, and friends compare the quality of care provided in the hospitals that agree to submit data on the quality of certain services they provide for certain conditions. This . . . not only helps you make good decisions about your health care, but also encourages hospitals to improve the quality of health care they provide." The site does not cover children's, psychiatric, rehabilitation, or long-term care hospitals.

***Joint Commission*** (formerly Joint Commission an Accreditation of Healthcare Organizations, or JCAHO)

*The Joint Commission*
*One Renaissance Boulevard*
*Oakbrook Terrace, IL 60181*
*Phone: 630-792-5000*
*www.jointcommission.org*

When choosing a hospital, make sure it is accredited by the Joint Commission. Visit *www.qualitycheck.org/consumer/searchQCR/aspx* to see how hospitals are viewed against national patient safety and quality standards. Determine how you want to conduct your search, fill in the relevant information, and follow the instructions. Note: the reports may take a very long time to load, even with a high-speed connection. Unless you want details, all you really need to know is whether the hospital is accredited.



### *MDLinx*

*1232 22nd Street NW*
*Suite 200*
*Washington, DC 20037*
*Phone: 202-293-2288*
*Fax: 202-293-1690*
*www.mdlinx.com/medical_newsletters.cfm*

This drug company-sponsored site does have advertising, but it also has some good material, especially about medical specialties. Click "Medical Newsletters" to view the list of specialties; there is also a newsletter aimed at patients. Uncheck the boxes to opt out of participating in market research (for honoraria) and receiving information from third parties about products or services.

### *Medem, Inc.*

*649 Mission Street, 2nd Floor*
*San Francisco, CA 94105*
*Phone: 877-926-3336*
*Fax: 415-644-3950*
*www.medem.com*

This physician-sponsored site connects physicians and patients online. Click "For Patients" to view options including (1) Create an iHealthrecord, (2) What is an iHealthrecord? (3) Sign up for education programs, (4) Start using online consultation, and (5) Find a physician on the Medem network.

***Medline Plus*** (a service of the U.S. National Library of Medicine and the National Institutes of Health)

*www.nlm.nih.gov/medlineplus/druginformation.html*

This site has excellent information on drugs, and since it is not commercially sponsored, it is free of ads and one-sided views. Enter the generic drug name if possible (i.e., phenytoin instead of Dilantan); otherwise, type the brand name into the "Search MedLine Plus" field on any page.

***Medscape Medical News***

*www.medscape.com*

Written by and for the medical community, this news board is good for research on conditions and research updates. Click on "Newsletters" and choose those of interest. (When the user is asked to indicate "position in medicine," one option is "consumer/other.")

***National Public Radio (NPR) Medical Newsletter***

*635 Massachusetts Avenue, NW*
*Washington, D.C. 20001*
*NPR Directory*
*Phone: 202-513-2000*
*Fax: 202-513-3329*
*www.npr.org/templates/topics/topic.php?topicId=1027*

This user-friendly site covers general news on health issues; users must sign in daily.

***Patient Advocate Foundation***

*700 Thimble Shoals Boulevard*
*Suite 200*
*Newport News, VA 23606*
*Phone: 800-532-5274*
*www.patientadvocate.org*

This national nonprofit "serves as an active liaison between the patient and their insurer, employer and/or creditors to resolve insurance, job retention and/or debt crisis matters relative to their diagnosis through case managers, doctors and attorneys."

***People's Medical Society***

*PO Box 868*
*Allentown, PA 18105-0868*
*Phone: 610-770-1670*
*www.peoplesmed.org*

This group's goals include: "Place previously unavailable information into the hands of ordinary people so that they can make informed decisions about their own health care; publish information designed to make every American a smart health care consumer; investigate and expose incidents of arrogance, incompetence and greed in organized medicine; protect the freedom to choose alternative providers of health care services; make the prevention of disease the top priority of American medicine; work toward creating an American health care system that is affordable, compassionate and centered around the needs of people."

***United Health Foundation***

*9900 Bren Road East*
*Minnetonka, MN 55343*
*www.unitedhealthfoundation.org*

This nonprofit private foundation's mission is "to support the health and medical decisions made by physicians, health professionals, community leaders and individuals that lead to better health outcomes and healthier communities."

***U.S. Living Will Registry***

*523 Westfield Avenue*
*PO Box 2789*
*Westfield, NJ 07091-2789*
*Phone: 800-LIV-WILL (800-548-9455)*
*Fax: 908-654-1919*
*www.uslivingwillregistry.com*

The registry's mission is "to promote the use of advance directives through educational programs, and to make people's health care choices available to their caregivers and families whenever and wherever they are needed, while maintaining the confidentiality of their information and documents." This site provides Living Will and Advance Directive information and storage and offers links to healthcare organizations for laypeople.

***Web MD Health***

*www.webmd.com*

By "trusted research organizations, manufacturers, and other leaders dedicated to treating and managing your health," this site covers topics such as diseases and conditions, symptoms, drugs and herbs, clinical trials, insurance plans, Medicare prescription benefits, and a medical "library."

***Your Personal Medical Assistant (PMA)***

*Strong Consulting*
*3 Castle Hill Court*
*Vallejo, CA 94591*
*Phone: 888-332-6297*
*www.anurseatyourside.com/pma.php*

The PMA system helps users consolidate, organize, and access their health-related documents and records. "Your PMA contains everything you need in one easy-to-find and easy-to-remember location . . . portable for easy reference during appointments." Available for a modest fee, including easy-to-use forms.

---

## Resources for Patient Advocates

***AARP*** (formerly American Association of Retired Persons)

*601 E Street NW*
*Washington, DC 20049*
*Phone: 888-OUR-AARP (888-687-2277)*
*www.research.aarp.org/health/ib35_medical_1.html*

A great general resource with a specific section on medical errors. Also provides information on end-of-life issues, wills, and estate planning.

***Agency for Healthcare Research and Quality***

*Office of Communications and Knowledge Transfer*
*540 Gaither Road, Suite 2000*
*Rockville, MD 20850*
*Phone: 301-427-1364*
*www.ahrq.gov/consumer/20tips.htm*

A part of the U.S. Department of Health and Human Services, this agency offers twenty tips to help prevent medical errors.

***Independent Production Fund***

*45 West 45th Street, Suite 808*
*New York, NY 10036*
*800-727-2470*
*www.whosedeathisitanyway.com*

This group produced "Whose Death Is It Anyway?" a documentary aired on PBS that "realistically explores the difficulties surrounding end-of-life decision making through five documentary segments that feature families sharing their own discussions and experiences."

***National Patient Safety Foundation***

*1120 MASS MoCA Way*
*North Adams, MA, 01247*
*Phone: 413-663-8900*
*Fax: 413-663-8905*
*www.npsf.org*

This nonprofit is an "indispensable resource for individuals and organizations committed to improving the safety of patients."

***Patients Are Powerful***

*PO Box 345*
*Penryn, CA 95663*
*Phone: 916-652-2293*
*Fax: 916-652-3427*
*www.patientsarepowerful.org*

Another nonprofit, this group "provides the reasons, steps and forms to empower patients."

***Today's Caregiver Magazine***

*Caregiver Media Group*
*3005 Greene Street*
*Hollywood, FL 33020*
*Phone: 800-829-2734*
*Fax: 954-893-1779*
*www.caregiver.com*

This site was developed by, for, and about caregivers. Includes a free online newsletter.

***wrongdiagnosis.com***

*www.wrongdiagnosis.com/mistakes/causes.htm*

This site was founded by patients, not doctors, so it is not medically sanctioned. It is written in everyday English and includes a good dictionary and a list of possible causes of medical mistakes.

---

## Palliative Care Resources

Fortunately, more hospitals are seeing the value of end-of-life transitional care and support, replacing the cold, white hospital setting with a kinder, gentler environment. Between 2000 and 2006, the number of hospitals providing palliative care almost doubled (from 632 to 1,240)—good news for the baby boomers approaching their senior years.[1]

The World Health Organization defines palliative care this way:

> Palliative care is an approach that improves the quality of life of patients and their families facing the problems associated with life-threatening illness, through the prevention and relief of suffering by means of early identification and impeccable

1 Robert Preidt, "Hospitals Continue to Implement Palliative Care Programs," *HealthDay News*, December 7, 2006, Medline Plus, http://www.healthfactsplus.com/print/news/fullstory_42326.html.

assessment and treatment of pain and other problems, physical, psychosocial and spiritual. Palliative care:

- provides relief from pain and other distressing symptoms
- affirms life and regards dying as a normal process
- intends neither to hasten or postpone death
- integrates the psychological and spiritual aspects of patient care
- offers a support system to help patients live as actively as possible until death
- offers a support system to help the family cope during the patients illness and in their own bereavement
- uses a team approach to address the needs of patients and their families, including bereavement counseling, if indicated
- will enhance quality of life, and may also positively influence the course of illness
- is applicable early in the course of illness, in conjunction with other therapies that are intended to prolong life, such as chemotherapy or radiation therapy, and includes those investigations needed to better understand and manage distressing clinical complications.[2]

Should this become the ultimate outcome of your patient's illness or injury, my prayers go with you. You may find these resources helpful.

***Caring Connections***

*National Hospice and Palliative Care Organization*
*1700 Diagonal Road, Suite 625*
*Alexandria, Virginia 22314*
*Phone: 703-837-1500*
*Fax: 703-837-1233 or 800-658-8898*
*www.caringinfo.org*

A program of the National Hospice and Palliative Care Organization (see next page), Caring Connections "provides free resources and information to help people make decisions about end-of-life care and services before a crisis;

2 World Health Organization, "WHO Definition of Palliative Care," http://www.who.int/cancer/palliative/definition/en.

helps people connect with the resources they need, when they need them; brings together community, state and national partners working to improve end-of-life care; spearheads a national consumer engagement campaign called 'It's About How You LIVE'; and provides free Advance Directives."



***growthhouse.org***

*Phone: 415-863-3045*
*www.growthhouse.org*

This site offers excerpts from the book *Handbook for Mortals* as well as *Fast Facts and Concepts,* a series of peer-reviewed, one-page outlines on end-of-life clinical topics for educators and clinicians.

***hospicecare.com***

*International Association for Hospice and Palliative Care*
*5535 Memorial Drive*
*Suite F—PMB 509*
*Houston TX 77007 USA*
*Phone: 866-374-2472*
*Fax: 713-880-2948*
*www.hospicecare.com/contact.htm*

This site offers wide-ranging material on hospice and palliative care services, including a newsletter and contact information for state-specific resources.

***Medscape Palliative Care Resource Center***

*www.medscape.com/resource/hospice*

Here you will find the latest clinical information on end-of-life care for adults and children, as well as information on supporting caregivers.

***National Hospice and Palliative Care Organization (NHPCO)***

*1700 Diagonal Road, Suite 625*
*Alexandria, Virginia 22314*
*Phone: 703- 837-1500*
*Fax: 703-837-1233*
*www.nhpco.org*

The largest nonprofit membership group of its kind in the United States, NHPCO is "committed to improving end of life care and expanding access to hospice care with the goal of profoundly enhancing quality of life for people dying in America and their loved ones." On this site you can "search for a care provider by name, city, state, or zip code and see the types of services they offer . . . search for vendors that specialize in the hospice and palliative care field; and find an end-of-life coalition in your community."

***Pain and Palliative Care Reporter***

*Bazelon Center for Mental Health Law*
*1101 Fifteenth Street NW*
*Suite 1212*
*Washington D.C. 20005*
*Phone: 202-467-5730*
*Fax: 202-223-0409*
*www.painlaw.org*

"The Palliative Care Reporter collects and disseminates legal materials and links that will assist attorneys and other advocates for patients who are in pain or who have a terminal illness; patients and families facing legal issues relating to withdrawing treatment at end of life; patients and families who have experienced poor pain management by their HMOs or doctors; doctors and other medical professionals who want to understand their rights and obligations under state and federal law; doctors or other medical persons who are under investigation for pain management prescription for legitimate pain patients."

## About This Book's Website

www.hospitalstayhandbook.com

Visit this book's website for more information and updates for patient advocates. Maintained by the author, the site includes the following:

- printable, reproducible "Care Team Notebook" pages (see Recommendation 11)
- medical terminology: an A–Z glossary of terms you may encounter in the hospital
- further resources: organizations, websites, publications, and more
- highlights of recent news on the U.S. healthcare system
- reviews of *Hospital Stay Handbook*
- background on Jari Holland Buck
- media kit

To contact the author, Jari Holland Buck, by mail, see the instructions on this book's copyright page. To reach her by e-mail, visit her own website. Follow the link found at www.hospitalstayhandbook.com.

# INDEX

For sample forms and legal documents, see this book's table of contents (they are not indexed here).

## Llewellyn Ordering Information

### Order Online:

Visit our website at www.llewellyn.com, select your books, and order them on our secure server.

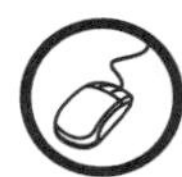

### Order by Phone:

- Call toll-free within the U.S. at 1-877-NEW-WRLD (1-877-639-9753). Call toll-free within Canada at 1-866-NEW-WRLD (1-866-639-9753)
- We accept VISA, MasterCard, and American Express

### Order by Mail:

Send the full price of your order (MN residents add 6.5% sales tax) in U.S. funds, plus postage & handling to:

**Llewellyn Worldwide**
**2143 Wooddale Drive, Dept. 978-0-7387-1224-6**
**Woodbury, MN 55125-2989**

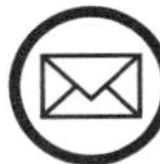

### Postage & Handling:

**Standard** (U.S., Mexico, & Canada). If your order is:
$24.99 and under, add $3.00
$25.00 and over, FREE STANDARD SHIPPING

AK, HI, PR: $15.00 for one book plus $1.00 for each additional book.

**International Orders** (airmail only):
$16.00 for one book plus $3.00 for each additional book

***Orders are processed within 2 business days.***
***Please allow for normal shipping time. Postage and handling rates subject to change.***

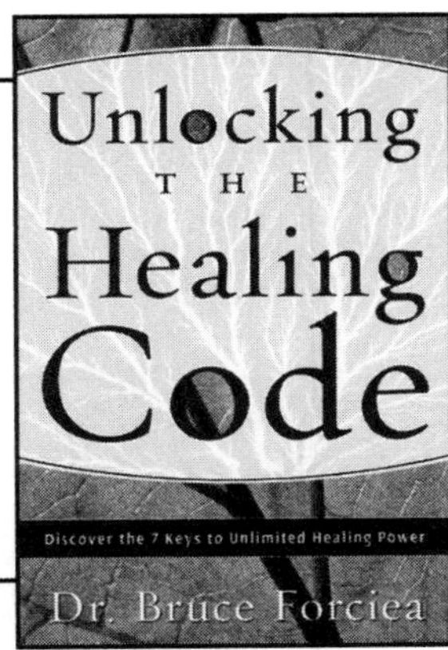


**Unlocking the Healing Code**

***Discover the 7 Keys to Unlimited Healing Power***

**Dr. Bruce Forciea**

Have you wondered why traditional medicine as well as herbs, homeopathy, and other alternative practices all work? They are all linked by a universal, mysterious field of energy that is alive with useful information. This healing information flows from the source to us across four channels, and anyone can learn how to activate these channels to heal injuries and recover from illness.

Bridging the gap between traditional and alternative healthcare, Dr. Bruce Forciea introduces seven keys to unlocking this unlimited healing power. His techniques, useful for both patients and practitioners, help you choose and apply complementary healing methodologies—such as creative visualization, vitamins, herbs, magnets, microcurrents, light, and chiropractics. True stories, including the author's own experience with recovering from chronic illness, highlight how numerous people have found relief using this groundbreaking program for healing.

**978-0-7387-1077-8**
**216 pp., 6 x 9** **$14.95**

## To Write to the Author

If you wish to contact the author or would like more information about this book, please write to the author in care of Llewellyn Worldwide and we will forward your request. Both the author and publisher appreciate hearing from you and learning of your enjoyment of this book and how it has helped you. Llewellyn Worldwide cannot guarantee that every letter written to the author can be answered, but all will be forwarded. Please write to:


Jari Holland Buck
℅ Llewellyn Worldwide
2143 Wooddale Drive, Dept. 978-0-7387-1224-6
Woodbury, MN 55125-2989, U.S.A.


Please enclose a self-addressed stamped envelope for reply, or $1.00 to cover costs. If outside U.S.A., enclose international postal reply coupon.

Many of Llewellyn's authors have websites with additional information and resources. For more information, please visit our website at:

www.llewellyn.com